CHAIR YOGA FOR SENIORS OVER 60

Improve Your Balance, Strength, and Mobility in Just 21 Days

Written by Industry Expert
ARTHUR HANSON

© **Copyright 2023 - All rights reserved.**

The content contained within this book may not be reproduced, duplicated, or transmitted without direct written permission from the author or the publisher.

Under no circumstances will any blame or legal responsibility be held against the publisher, or author, for any damages, reparation, monetary loss, injury, or health related issue due to the information contained within this book, either directly or indirectly.

Legal Notice:

This book is copyright protected. It is only for personal use. You cannot amend, distribute, sell, use, quote or paraphrase any part, or the content within this book, without the consent of the author or publisher.

Disclaimer Notice:

Please note the information contained within this document is for educational and entertainment purposes only. All effort has been executed to present accurate, up to date, reliable, complete information. No warranties of any kind are declared or implied. Readers acknowledge that the author is not engaged in the rendering of legal, financial, medical or professional advice. The content within this book has been derived from various sources. Please consult a licensed professional before attempting any techniques outlined in this book.

By reading this document, the reader agrees that under no circumstances is the author responsible for any losses, direct or indirect, that are incurred as a result of the use of the information contained within this document, including, but not limited to, errors, omissions, or inaccuracies.

CONTENTS

	Introduction	1
Chapter 1	What You Need to Know Before You Get Started	8
Chapter 2	Your First Chair Yoga Poses	33
Chapter 3	Standing and Floor Based Yoga Poses	64
Chapter 4	Morning Chair Yoga Routine	85
Chapter 5	Evening Chair Yoga Routine	98
Chapter 6	Beginner Chair Yoga Program: Day 1 - 7	114
Chapter 7	Intermediate Chair Yoga Program: Day 8 - 14	139
Chapter 8	Advanced Chair Yoga Program: Day 15 - 21	160
	Conclusion	181
	References	184

CHAIR YOGA FOR SENIORS OVER 60

INTRODUCTION

"Yoga is not a religion. It is a science of well-being, science of youthfulness, science of integrating body, mind, and soul."

- AMIT RAY

Yoga is an ancient practice that has been utilized for over 5000 years. The basic poses, exercises, and stretches were developed to help treat stress, anxiety, and many everyday aches and pains. Even though yoga has been around for thousands of years, it is still relevant today, enabling its practitioners to gain huge benefits such as increased muscular strength, improved flexibility and balance, and improved posture. All of these benefits can be achieved from practicing the positions and movements for as little as 5 to 10 minutes per day.

Yoga is great for everyone. Whether you are an avid exercise enthusiast who has years of experience under your belt or you have never hit the gym before, there are poses and stretches made just for you when it comes to yoga. And when you learn about all the great benefits that come with it, the only thing that you'll wonder is why you didn't start sooner!

The Benefits of Chair Yoga

Whether you decide to spend five minutes or an hour per day practicing your chair yoga poses, you will quickly see how it will significantly improve the quality of your life, allowing you to always be at your absolute best. Some of the mental and physical benefits that participants will enjoy from their very first session include:

- Improved balance, flexibility, and strength.
- Relief from chronic back pain without medications.
- Eased arthritis symptoms.
- Keeping your heart healthy by helping to reduce body inflammation and stress.
- Reduced anxiety by relaxing your mind and body, making falling into a restful sleep easier.
- Increased energy levels and improved mood.
- Managing your stress and living your best life.

Overall, chair yoga helps you slow down from all the hustle and bustle that goes on in our modern world. It promotes self-care as you learn more about your body and how it moves. It may seem silly to do the poses when you start, but as you encourage the positive flow of energy through your body, you will quickly see what a massive difference it will make.

INTRODUCTION

Why Should I Start Practicing Chair Yoga?

Do you struggle with pain in your daily life, finding it hard to get many routine tasks done without discomfort? Is your balance not as good as it used to be, and have you noticed your posture is not as strong and straight as you'd like? Does pain or discomfort negatively affect your self-confidence and your quality of sleep? Do you feel like you can't live life to the fullest because of limitations on your mobility and stability?

If you are like many of my clients, you will find that at least one of the above scenarios matches your current situation. Taking a little time each day to improve yourself will make your quality of life soar through the roof. Your current experience level does not matter. Instead, put your focus on being consistent with your practice for the next 21 days and let the yoga do the rest.

In this guide, we will work together to answer all your questions and discover precisely how chair yoga will improve your life in as little as 10 minutes per day!

What if Pain and Flexibility Limit My Movements?

You may have struggled with mobility over the past few years and haven't been able to stay as active as you would like due to joint or muscle discomfort. Whether that's holding you back at home, out and about, or at the gym, the feeling of "that's just the way that it is" doesn't need to be a part of your vocabulary. So many people live with pain and discomfort that could be ironed out with the right exercise routine. With that in mind, there's no need to just let something that can usually so easily be resolved slow you down and make it hard to keep up with all the activities that you love.

If you've been trying to find a low-impact but progressive program that can improve your flexibility and increase your pain-free mobility, chair yoga is exactly what you've been looking for. When used correctly, it is the key to helping you stay active as you age, even if you struggle with joint pain or if you have never worked out before. Whether you can practice while standing or if you need to sit down, the yoga poses and programs in this book have been designed in such a way that they can be modified and adapted to work for you.

In this guidebook, we will look at yoga positions with variations ranging from beginner to advanced so that you can get the most out of your chair yoga programs, even if you're new to it. To begin with I have included programs to help you work on both dynamic and static stretching to improve your base flexibility. I then take you through routines with the goal of getting you up and active in the morning, and helping you to unwind and relax in the evening. I have also included a progressive yoga program suitable for all levels that takes you from a total beginner to intermediate to advanced, all in just 21 days.

How I Can Help

As the author of this book, I am uniquely qualified to help guide you on your chair yoga journey by ensuring that you get the very best results that will keep you living a healthy life of independence.

INTRODUCTION

With more than 20 years of experience as a one-on-one personal trainer and yoga instructor, as well as a highly qualified sports therapist and injury rehab specialist, I have been lucky enough to work with thousands of clients of all ages to work toward improving and protecting their overall health, fitness and physical abilities while achieving the goals that they never thought were possible!

Whether my clients are looking to improve their balance and flexibility, lose weight, gain strength, or even if their focus is directed toward reducing the aches and pains that they have. I have worked closely with them and have come up with workout plans that speak to their goals, and through this, I have tried and tested methods that work!

The good news in this is that by applying my 20-plus years experience as an exercise professional and sports rehab specialist, I have been able to create workouts that target the specific movement patterns in the correct order to help rebalance your body, strengthen your muscles, and reduce (or totally eradicate!) pain where possible, all while moving you towards the new, fitter, and healthier you.

Over the years, I have also developed a deep love and appreciation for yoga. While some of the poses may seem quite simple, they can work incredibly well for a host of different conditions for individuals of any age. Whether I'm working with a 20-year-old athlete recovering from a sports-related shoulder injury, a 40-year-old learning to walk pain-free again after knee surgery, or someone in their late 60s with an aching lower back and arthritic pain, combining yoga with my other exercise principles can be genuinely life-changing for them.

You Can Learn Chair Yoga at Any Age!

In this fully illustrated guidebook, we will cover everything you need to take you at your own pace, from a chair yoga beginner by looking at basic posture exercises and positions right up to being able to work through advanced chair yoga programs. Beyond thinking of this as just another book of exercises, together we will be taking a look at exactly how following these carefully constructed programs for just 21 days, even if you start with as little as 10 minutes a day, will benefit your body, your health, and your mind.

Inside, you will learn:

- The benefits of chair yoga and why the best time to get started is today.
- How to use the correct breathing techniques while practicing chair yoga to improve your sessions, and how it will help reduce stress and anxiety.
- Learn the key beginner poses to get you started right away, no matter your experience level, flexibility, or age.
- Why chair yoga is so beneficial in the morning and which simple and effective stretches to use to get you going.
- The benefits of an evening chair yoga routine to help you relax and fall into a restful sleep.
- Exactly how to progress from a beginner to an advanced level, starting with some easy poses to get you going.
- An effective 21-day routine, suitable for all skill levels.

INTRODUCTION

Yoga may have been around for more than 5000 years, but the application is still one of the most effective forms of low-impact exercise today. With my experience, the proven information in this guidebook, and a little practice on your part, you will be able to achieve and maintain the active life of independence you want!

1

WHAT YOU NEED TO KNOW BEFORE YOU GET STARTED

"A yogi measures the span of life by the number of breaths, not by the number of years."

- SWAMI SIVANANDA

The idea of hitting the gym and comparing yourself to younger athletes while you work on your flexibility may make you break out into a cold sweat, especially if you are in pain or discomfort. Chair yoga is a great solution. With simple stretches and deep breathing, you can improve your flexibility and feel almost immediate relief. And all from the comfort of your home! To help you get started with chair yoga, we will lay out some basics to help you get the most out of your practice.

Why Correct Breathing is Important in Yoga

As you've probably already gathered, good form and stretching are both important when you practice chair yoga, but what can often be overlooked is learning how to breathe with the movements to ensure that you get the most from each pose. I would like for you to think of how you breathe as an integral part of your form while you run through your programs.

When we think about and consciously control our breathing, rather than just letting it happen automatically, we can activate a separate part of the brain. Unconscious breathing, which is automatic, is controlled by the medulla oblongata. The cerebral cortex controls conscious breathing.

Consciously breathing sends impulses from the cortex to the areas of the brain that impact your emotions. It can relax and balance your mood while controlling your emotions if done right. Controlling your breathing and focusing on the emotions that matter allows you to have total control.

Let's look at an example. What do you notice about your breathing when you're anxious or upset? It is often elevated, with short and frequent bursts occurring the whole time. Your adrenaline is pumping when this happens, and you are in a heightened state of arousal until the breathing slows down. You can replicate this process. Take a few minutes and force your breathing to pick up. You should notice your heart rate goes up, and you are more alert.

This works the other way too. What do you notice about your breathing when you feel calm and relaxed? It is no longer quick and shallow like before but often slow and steady. You take deep, cleansing breaths that make you feel amazing, slow down the heart rate, and release all the tension.

This is just an example of what chair yoga can do for you. You learn how to control your breathing, slow it down, and bring on the relaxation you need. For those who struggle with stress, anger, or anxiety, just slowing down your breathing can be enough to help you calm down and feel better than before. Yoga has many poses, whether sitting, standing, or lying down, that ask for deep, controlled breathing. This is often enough to relax you and reduce the stress and anxiety.

How to Yoga Breathe

Yoga breathing is slightly different from how you breathe during your normal daily activities. During yoga, you must slow yourself down and focus on taking deep breaths all the way down to the stomach, allowing it to fully expand before letting it release along with all the stress and toxins from your body simultaneously.

Some of the simple steps you can use to accomplish the peace and calm you need during yoga are as follows:

- Find a quiet spot where you can be alone while you practice. Get comfortable. Relax your body and bring all your focus to your breathing.

WHAT YOU NEED TO KNOW BEFORE YOU GET STARTED

- Take a moment to analyze your current breathing pattern. Don't try to change or control anything yet. Let it come naturally and determine what is going on.
- When you are ready, take a deep breath in through the nose, letting your stomach expand as much as you comfortably can.
- When reaching the peak of your inhale, feel your rib cage expand. You should notice that your shoulders and collarbones also begin to elevate.
- Slowly and gently start exhaling out of your mouth. Feel the release travel down your body, feeling your shoulders and collarbones release, followed by your upper chest, middle chest, and then the stomach.
- If possible, try to hold each breath for three to five seconds after exhaling and then repeat. Don't force it. This should feel natural and will improve with practice.

Run through these steps now for a few minutes before we move on to help lock it into your mind, ready for later. You should adjust to the slower breathing technique and have a chance to feel a wave of calm and relaxation come over you. For this exercise, you should sit comfortably with your back straight and your hands in your lap.

Now that you have the hang of it, you can easily transfer these breathing techniques to the yoga poses we will be practicing shortly.

Why Should I Warm Up Before Starting?

Even though yoga may not require pumping iron, running around, or getting a tough sweat on, you still need to take the time to warm up before you begin your session. This helps mobilize the joints and loosen up the muscles to prevent injury and get the blood flowing so you can get the most out of your yoga routine. Some of the reasons to consider warming up before you begin yoga include:

- Improves your blood flow: A proper warm up before practicing yoga will increase circulation to your muscles. It can ensure your muscles have the essential energy to hold and sustain the different poses.
- Improves flexibility: Flexibility is important, especially as we age. Chair yoga can help improve your flexibility naturally and safely. You can build endurance and become more flexible as you practice yoga more often, but a good warm up and stretch before your workout can also make a difference. The correct sequence of stretching improves flexibility quicker than anything else.
- Minimizes risk of injury: Without a good warm up, it is more likely you will become prone to injuries during the session. This can include straining a muscle or pushing a joint too far too quickly. Even just a few minutes of stretching before you begin yoga will make a difference to both muscle and joint health.

Your warm up does not have to be tough or take long. Starting with simple neck rotations, side tilts, and shoulder rolls will do wonders to prepare your body for exercise. You can even reach for your toes or move around in a gentle walk. The key here is simply to get your body moving for a few minutes before starting your routine.

The Differences Between Static and Dynamic Stretching

There are two main types of stretching: dynamic and static. Dynamic stretching is when you actively move the muscles and joints in and out of the stretch position under control, usually for ten to twelve repetitions. The movement you do while dynamically stretching mimics the activity you are warming up for while preparing your muscles and joints and will improve your body's performance.

Then there is static stretching, where you hold a controlled stretch position, usually between 30 to 90 seconds, enough so that you can feel your muscles lengthening without feeling pain. If you have ever sat on the ground with your legs straight out in front of you and reached for your toes, then this is an example of a static stretch.

In short, dynamic stretching is best used to prepare your body for physical activity, which is why they are great to use in a warm up. Static stretching is usually considered more of a cool down after exercise to help the body relax and recover, and should only be used once your muscles have been properly warmed up.

Dynamic Stretches to Try

As mentioned before, dynamic stretching helps loosen up your muscles, preparing you for exercise through movement. Here are some examples that I recommend:

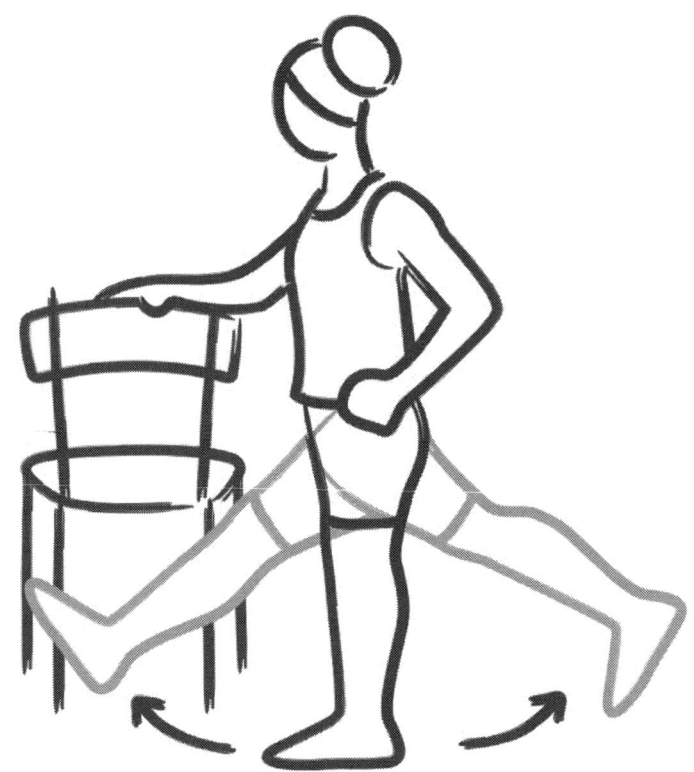

Leg Pendulums (Hamstrings and Hip Flexors)

- Place one hand on a wall or hold the back of a chair for balance.
- Stand on one leg (keeping it straight).
- Swing the other leg (also straight) forward and backward 10 to 12 times.

WHAT YOU NEED TO KNOW BEFORE YOU GET STARTED

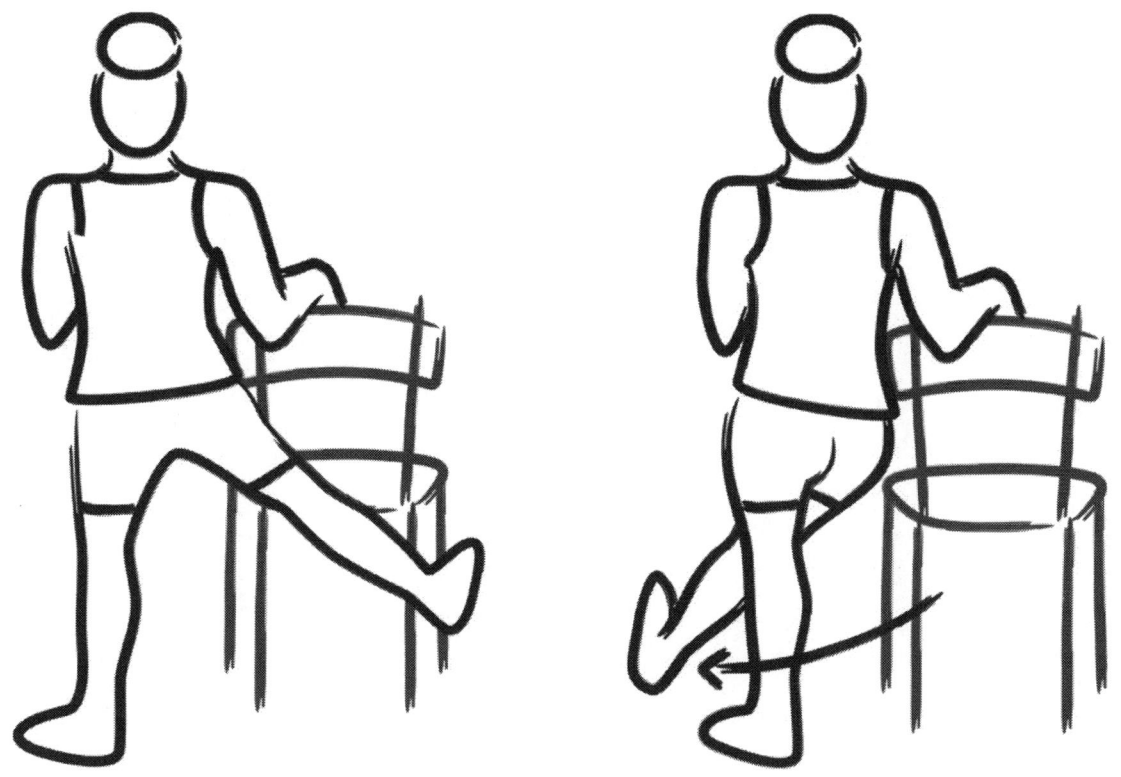

Leg Pendulums (Adductors and Abductors)

- Now, turn to face the wall or chair and use both hands to balance.
- Using the same concept, swing one leg across your body in a side-to-side motion.
- When dynamic stretching like this, always hold onto something for balance and swing in a smooth and gentle motion.

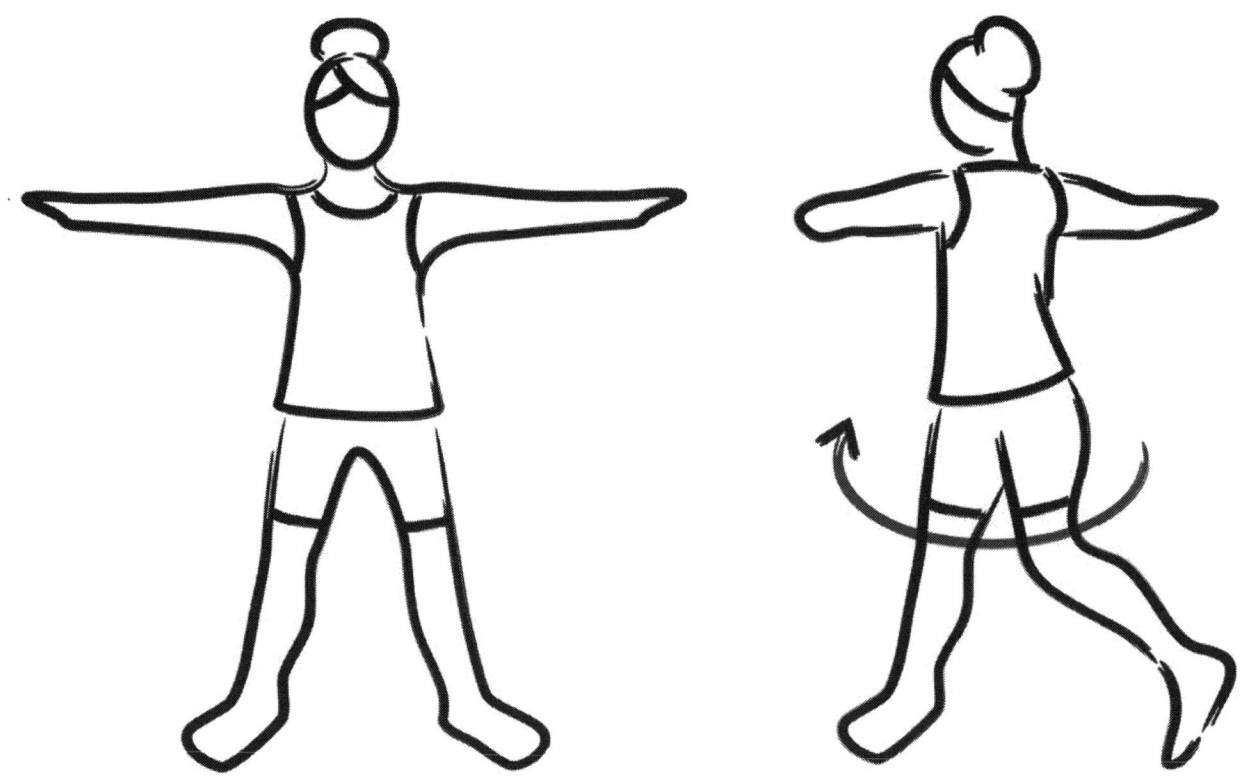

Trunk Twists

- Standing with your feet apart or sitting down on a chair with knees bent and feet on the ground.
- Keep your torso as upright as possible with your arms straight out to the sides at shoulder height.
- Slowly twist the torso to the right, allowing your arms to lead your body around, feeling a gentle stretch in your middle.
- Hold for a moment and then gently mimic the movement to the opposite side.
- Repeat this gentle 'swinging' action for 8 to 10 repetitions in each direction.

WHAT YOU NEED TO KNOW BEFORE YOU GET STARTED

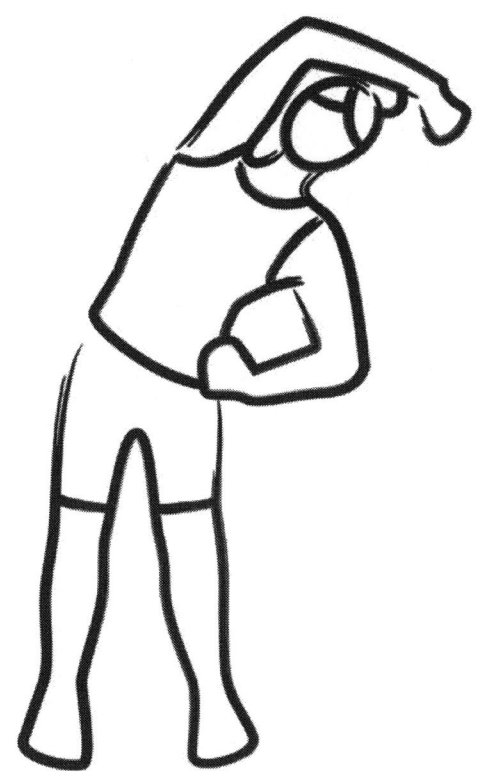

Side Bends

- Stand with your feet hip distance apart or sit in a chair with knees bent and feet on the ground.
- Bend the right arm so the right hand is to the right side of the head.
- Allow the left arm to hang to the side.
- Take a breath in, and as you exhale, bend at the waist to lower the left arm to the floor.
- Pull the right elbow back to feel the stretch. Breathe in and return to an upright position.
- Repeat on the other side.

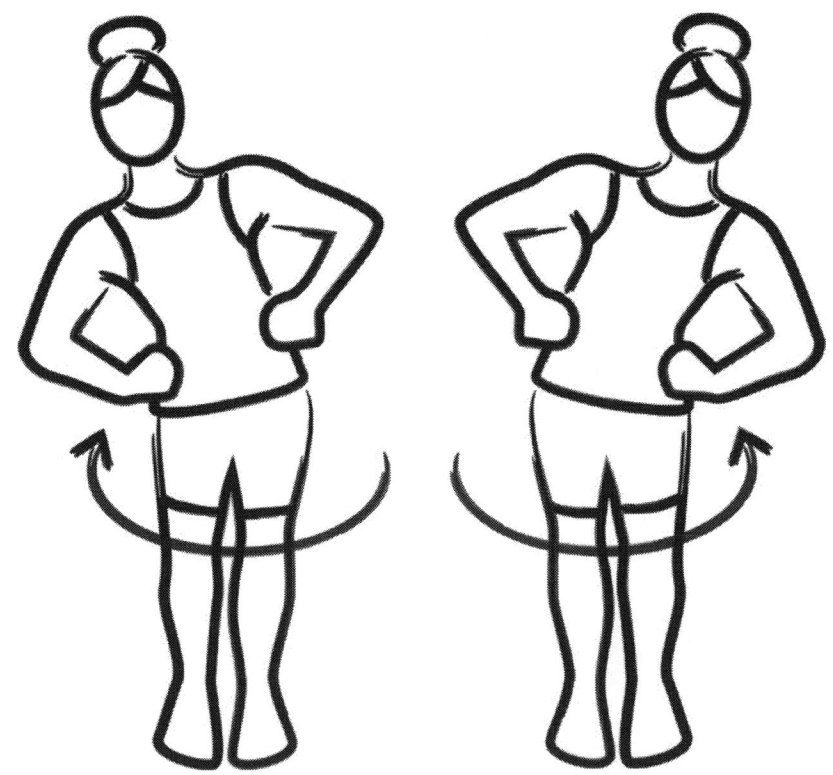

Hip Circles

- Stand upright with your feet shoulder distance apart.
- Keeping your legs straight, circle your hips in a clockwise motion. You're looking to mobilize rather than push here, so keep the action gentle and smooth.
- After 10-12 rotations, stop and repeat in the opposite direction.

WHAT YOU NEED TO KNOW BEFORE YOU GET STARTED

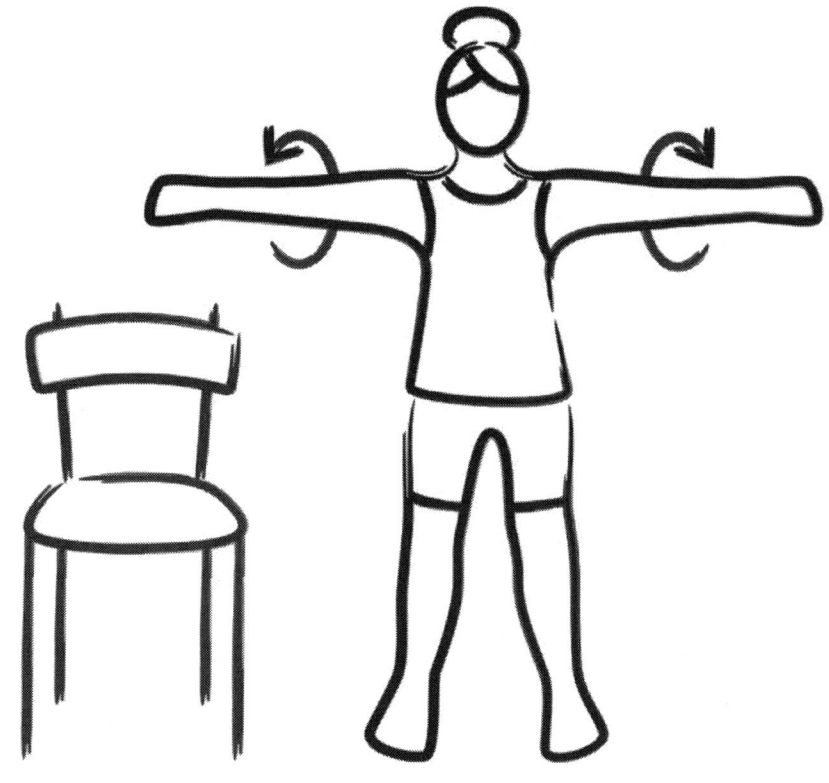

Arm Circles

- Hold the arms out parallel to the shoulders.
- Rotate them in small circles forward for 30 counts.
- Now reverse the action and go backward for 30 counts.
- Once the arm muscles feel warm, make the arm circles larger.

While movement is an essential part of dynamic stretching, take your time to practice each dynamic stretch, and if something doesn't feel right, stop the movement and try the next one. You should never combine any of these dynamic stretches with ballistic (bouncing or disjointed) motions. The idea is to go at your own pace to properly prepare yourself for the programs ahead. Over the coming weeks, as your fitness, flexibility, and balance improve, you can gradually increase the intensity. Until then, listen to your body and work at a rate that works for you.

Static Stretches to Try

After your body is warm or at the end of a yoga session, holding a static stretch is a great way to further develop your range and mobility, as well as help your body cool down. Here are some simple static stretches you can use after your chair yoga routine:

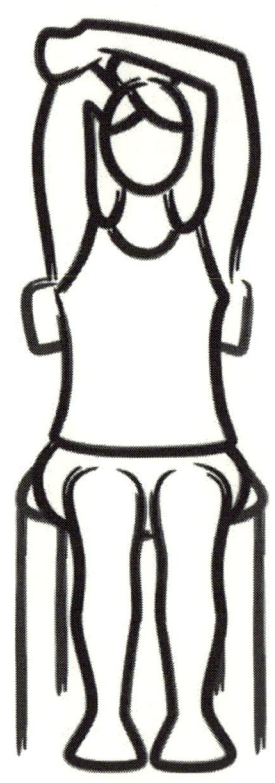

Overhead Triceps Stretch

- Sitting or standing, keep the feet hip-width apart and roll the shoulders back and down.

WHAT YOU NEED TO KNOW BEFORE YOU GET STARTED

- Reach the right arm to the ceiling, bending the elbow so the right palm is down to your back.
- Bring the left hand up and gently push the right elbow down. Hold for 20 to 30 seconds.
- Switch the arms around and repeat on the other side.

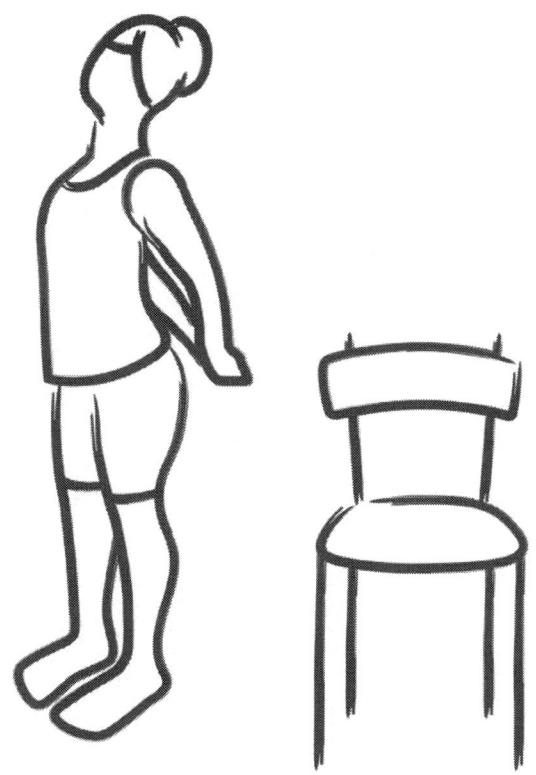

Biceps Stretch

- Stand or sit up straight with both hands behind your back, interlaced at the base of the spine.
- Face your palms down and straighten your arms.
- Lift your chest and try to create a space between your hands and your body to increase the stretch in the shoulders and biceps.
- Hold for 30 seconds and release. Repeat 2 or 3 times.

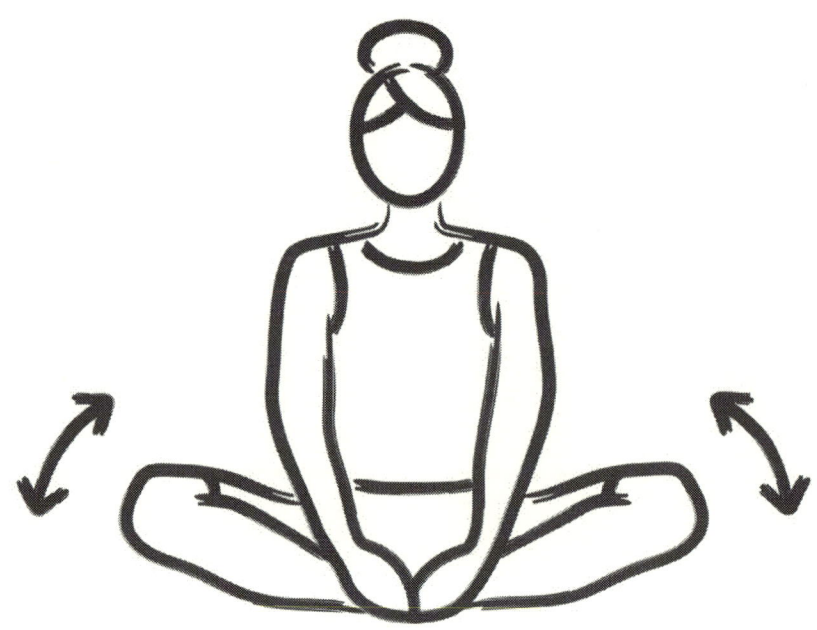

Seated Butterfly Stretch

- Sit on the floor, keeping the back straight, and draw your tummy in a little to help keep your abs engaged.
- With bent knees, place the soles of the feet together to the front, allowing your knees to fall out to the sides.
- If you can, hold onto your feet and gently pull the heels towards your hips. Let the knees relax and hang towards the floor.
- Breathing deeply, hold the pose for up to 30 seconds.

WHAT YOU NEED TO KNOW BEFORE YOU GET STARTED

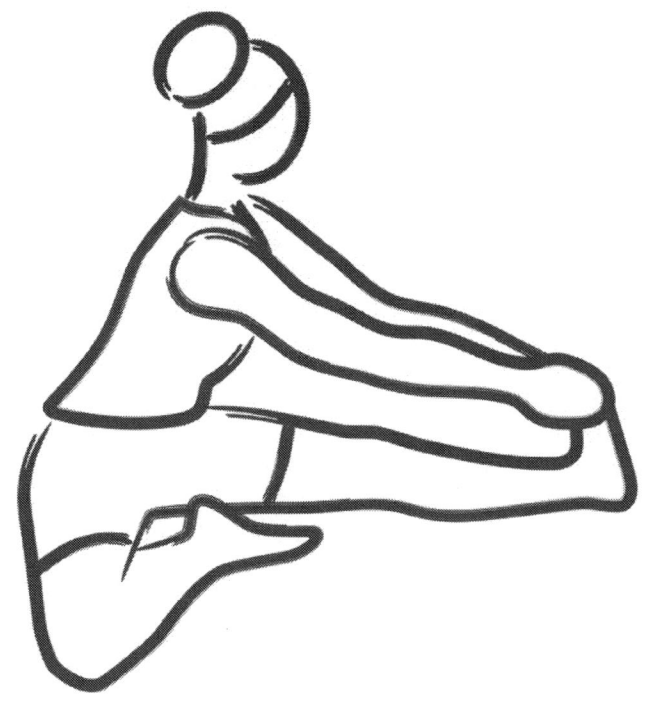

Head to Knee Forward Bend

- Sit down on the ground, extending your left leg straight out in front, and bring the sole of your right foot to the inside of the thigh.
- Inhale and lift your arms up to the ceiling. Exhale as you lengthen the spine, hinge at the hips, and tip your body forward toward the outstretched leg.
- Rest your hands as far forward as you comfortably can, either on the foot, legs, or floor. Hold this pose to stretch for a minute.
- Release and repeat on the opposite side.

With all of these static and dynamic stretch examples, it's about listening to your body and going at your own pace. To get lasting results, it's not about going as hard as possible from day one! Only by practicing consistently over the coming weeks will you see the improvements to your range, technique, balance, and overall skill level that you want.

Remember to Set Some Goals

Before you embark on your chair yoga journey, I recommend that you set at least one personal goal. Having a target to focus on will motivate you to keep moving toward your desired outcome each day. If you just get started without any goals, it is far more difficult to stay on track with your daily practice, which can end up limiting your results.

When setting a goal, think about where you currently are and then think about where you want to be. Your goal needs to be tough enough that you will need to work to reach it, but not so tough that you have no chance of achieving success. Break your goal down into bite-sized pieces (I call these 'daily goals') to help you know what little actions you need to do each day to form a new lifestyle habit.

Forming a habit does not need to take long. It just requires a little bit of consistency and dedication. You can't expect outstanding results if you only dedicate yourself to one or two days. You should choose an amount of time that allows you to get used to the new endeavor, but not so long that it seems overwhelming!

I recommend setting a goal for 21 days when starting out with chair yoga. This is just enough time to form a habit and integrate chair yoga into your daily routine without it taking so long that you end up feeling overwhelmed and want to stop. When you have completed your first two weeks, you will notice significant improvements in flexibility, your stress levels, your muscular and joint tightness or pain, your mood, and overall health. Once you've seen what chair yoga can do for you and how simply it will slot into your daily life, staying motivated to keep practicing will feel easy.

The Importance of Good Form and Focus

While the poses are important, you should take the time to focus on your form. These are sometimes even more important than the actual poses themselves. If you have poor form, you increase your risk of injury, and your results will take longer to achieve. The right focus, along with proper posture, will help you get the most out of your chair yoga practice.

Let's start with the basics of good form in chair yoga. Sitting with a good, straight back, with your feet flat on the floor and hands in your lap, is a good place to start. Add a pillow underneath you or to support the small of your back if your posture feels strained as you work to strengthen those muscles.

Each pose will require a different form, so pay close attention to what is recommended and how your body feels along the way. If something feels off balance or hurts, then you are either pushing too far or not maintaining the strong posture that you need.

Some things to keep in mind when it comes to maintaining good form in yoga include:

- Keep the back straight. Whether you are sitting, lying down, or standing, your back should be straight, not curved, to allow for lengthening and fewer issues with pain.
- Only go as far as you can handle pain-free. It's good to push yourself a little, but don't make anything painful to complete.
- Focus on the breathing. Your breathing should be easy. If it is labored or you find a position that makes it difficult to breathe in, this is a sign that something is not working well. If this does happen, please stop, reset, and try again. If a pose still isn't working for you, please skip over it in your workout and come back to it another day.

Chair yoga is all about focus. You need to focus on a number of things to make sure you get the most out of each pose. For example, **as we discussed earlier**, you need to focus on your breathing and make sure your stretches are right for the pose you choose. Some people find focusing on a mantra or sound can help clear their minds and prevent their thoughts from wandering. You can also focus on an object in front of you to help with balance and coordination as you get better with the movements.

As you perfect your focus, you will find that this new skill can translate to other aspects of your life. For example, when there is a stressful situation at work or home, you can use some of the focus from yoga to calm down your breathing and clear your mind before making an important decision.

When to Push Yourself and When to Take It Easy

This is one of the hardest things to gauge when starting your yoga journey. You want to make sure to push yourself a little, trying a new pose or pushing just a little further, but you also need to be gentle on your body and not go so hard that you cause injury or lose motivation. Finding that balance can take time and a good understanding of your own body.

On most days, you should push your body a bit and see how far you can confidently take the pose and how much you can improve over the day before. You don't want to go so hard that you cause pain and strain to the muscles to an extreme, but a little burn is not a bad thing. When you feel ready to push on, try the next level on a pose or implement a new pose that may have been too difficult previously.

Of course, there will be those days that you feel worn out and your muscles ache. On those days, it's fine to take a step back and relax. Do some of the relaxation poses and just stretch out the body. This can help relieve the tension to keep you on track. Interestingly, your muscles develop from your training as you recover and not while you train, so with that in mind, give your body some extra time when it needs it.

How to Progress Your Chair Yoga Routine

The goal, of course, when you begin any exercise program is to see steady, continuous progress. Whether your goals are to increase your strength, improve your balance and mobility, improve your posture and flexibility, or if it's to simply become more active and build your self-confidence, you should feel as though you're always moving forward. I have given some ideas for you to consider to help maximize your results:

- **Always warm up:** Warming your muscles and joints up before beginning your yoga routine is vital and should never be overlooked!
- **Practice makes progress:** Make chair yoga a part of your daily routine and see yourself progress. Even as little as ten minutes a day is enough to move you toward your health and fitness goals. The more time you can devote to the poses and the work, the faster you will improve.
- **Avoid the comparison to others:** Your journey is all your own. The only comparison you should make is when you look at where you started compared with where you are now.
- **Be consistent:** When it comes to chair yoga (just like learning any other skill), consistency is key. You will get better results by practicing for 10 minutes each day than you will from a mammoth 70-minute session once per week!
- **Never force it:** We talked about the importance of pushing your body a bit when you enter into a pose to see whether you are ready to progress to the next level. Pushing is not a bad thing, but never force a movement or a pose. If it hurts or something doesn't feel right, then stop!
- **Remember your breathing technique:** Of course, in yoga, the poses are important, but so is the breathing! Keep up the deep, cleansing breathing to ensure that you will be able to fully

oxygenate your muscles, remove any negativity, and keep your body going strong for your whole routine.

- **Never skip the relaxation:** After completing your yoga routine, take the time to stretch and relax. This is an easy step to skip over, but it can make all the difference to your recovery and results.
- **Pick a routine that works for you:** Take a look at your current schedule, your fitness level, and other factors in your day, and then pick a chair yoga routine that works for you. We will discuss the benefits of chair yoga both in the morning and the evening later in the book. If you can do both, that is amazing. If not, pick the one that works best for your routine.

Your progress is all your own. As long as you are moving forward and see changes in your flexibility and strength, then you are doing an amazing job.

The Mind/Muscle Connection

Yoga is all about fully connecting your mind with the body to gain total control over your muscles and movements while giving it the stretch it deserves. The mind/muscle connection requires you to focus on the muscle or muscle group you want to improve as you move rather than just going through the motions and not feeling what you're supposed to. If you just sit down on the chair and go through the motions without thinking about what each pose is targeting, your results will stall.

Don't get me wrong, repeating movements and poses without focusing on your mind/muscle connection will still provide benefits (especially as a beginner) but ultimately won't give you the full results your effort deserves, which is why I always encourage everyone that I'm working with to work on it from the first day of their program, as this will start to instill the good habits that will become second nature pretty quickly.

Some simple ways to help you improve your mind/muscle connection are to slow down your movements, warm up the specific muscles you need before the main workout, bracing (contracting) to target muscles during the pose or at the end of each repetition, and visualizing the area that needs to stretch can be enough to connect the mind to the muscle and get better results.

Your chair yoga workout does not need to be long. You can put in the extra effort to focus on the muscle groups in your routine to connect the mind to the body for fifteen to twenty minutes a day. Chase the pump and focus on the muscle rather than going through the motions and missing all the benefits of chair yoga.

Key Takeaways

- Chair yoga is a fantastic workout that reduces stress and anxiety and improves focus.
- Chair yoga is suitable for all fitness levels, has been proven to greatly reduce joint and muscular pain, and best of all, doesn't need a gym membership or any fancy training equipment.
- Correct breathing technique is an important part of chair yoga. Among other health benefits, when you focus on sustaining a pose, how you breathe helps to control your heart rate and your enjoyment of the feeling.

- Always make sure you take the time to stretch dynamically before beginning your chair yoga routine. It may not be as intense as other forms of exercise, but stretching can help keep you safe and injury-free.
- Consider setting some simple goals. This will help keep you focused on what you want and what you need to do, and will ensure that you see results in no time.
- Learning how to listen to your body and form that important mind/muscle connection can improve so many aspects of your life.

Practicing chair yoga can be done any time of the day that is most convenient to you, but there are many benefits to waking up and starting your day with this activity. In the next chapter, we will take a look at the simple steps to start a morning chair yoga routine and the benefits of implementing this practice into your day.

FREE BONUS:
WARM UP EXERCISES CHART AND FULL AUDIOBOOK

I think that it can feel quite tricky to practice new exercises while holding a book open on the right page. To help with this, I have created video guides and a chart with each of the warm up exercises pictured in this chapter enlarged and printable to make your life easier.

I have also included the full audiobook version of this book so that you can listen along as you run through your movements. I'm a big believer in giving as much as possible to each and every one of my awesome clients to ensure that they can get the absolute most out of their exercise programs.

Go to your internet browser and type in bit.ly/chair-yoga-free and I'll get them to you.

You can also scan the QR Code below with your cell phone camera and tap the little link that appears if you find that easier.

All the bonuses I offer are extremely helpful and totally free!

2

YOUR FIRST CHAIR YOGA POSES

"Yoga teaches us to cure what need not be endured and endure what cannot be cured."

- B.K.S IYENGAR

Now that we've talked about how to stretch your body both dynamically and statically, and you have the basic concepts of what chair yoga is all about, let's dive straight into your first chair yoga poses. The awesome thing about chair yoga is that you can gain all the health benefits of regular yoga without having to worry about your current balance, flexibility, or core strength. The movements and poses are all designed to be progressive, meaning that you can modify and adapt them to suit you, whether you're a total beginner or already at an advanced level.

These chair yoga poses mimic the ones you can use while standing or lying down while fully supporting you so that you are able to stay in full control whether this is your first or fiftieth time experiencing yoga. Just because these are the first chair yoga poses that we are learning together doesn't mean they are the easiest. I have chosen them to give you a good idea of what your chair yoga journey is going to look like.

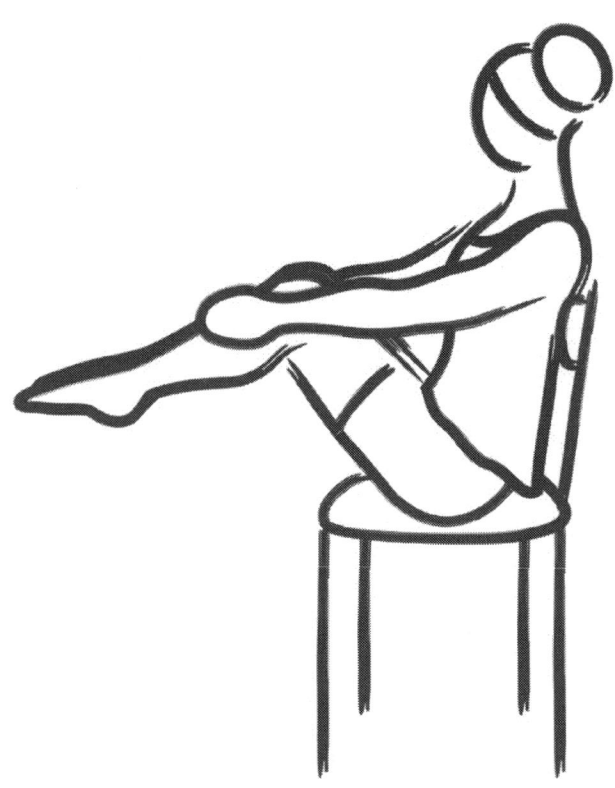

Boat

The goal of the Boat Pose is to bring the arms up and out, using them as a 'downward driver' (in other words, using your arms to activate and load your muscles lower down in your body). Always remember that if you need some extra support at the beginning, then leave your palms on the ground to help. Lift the legs up as high as you can, slowly working up to a 45-degree angle.

Please follow the teaching points below:

- Sit in an upright posture on your chair away from the backrest. Hold onto either side of the chair's seat with your hands, and slowly extend and raise your legs with bent knees in front of you.
- As you raise your legs, slowly lean back until your upper back is upon the chair's backrest. You should now feel your core muscles engage. As a little side note, you'll hear me talk about your core muscles quite a bit in this book. I want you to think of your core as your 'natural weightlifting belt' that wraps around your waist; you can 'activate' it by simply drawing your belly button in towards your spine with a slight bracing of your abs.
- Keep your hands holding onto the seat until you feel confident to move on to the next part. Remember that if you are a beginner, starting off with a slight leg raise, a short hold, and then returning to the start position is great. When you feel ready to progress, continue to the next teaching points.
- Inhale and bring your knees up towards your chest, stopping when the thighs reach a 45-degree angle to the ground. When you feel confident with your form and core strength, try to gradually extend your legs to further engage your muscles and increase the difficulty.
- Extend your arms out in front of you, with them parallel to the floor. Hold for up to 30 seconds, and then return to your starting position.

As mentioned above, as you gain core strength, you will slowly be able to extend your legs out further in front of you. This will increase the difficulty and help you improve your strength by gradually increasing the load through your body.

Notes:

Remember that with all exercise programs, your training form always comes first. Exercising with the correct form means that you will target the parts of your body that you're supposed to, which ultimately accelerates your results.

So, in the case of the Boat Pose, if you start off gripping the seat and you manage to hold the pose for 3 seconds for each repetition, pat yourself on the back because that's an excellent way to begin. As you progress and your core strength improves (which it will pretty quickly if you exercise consistently!), you can increase the difficulty of the pose, the number of repetitions, and the length of time that you hold each repetition.

This advice applies to all exercises and all training programs. I just thought that it's a good place to mention it.

Anyway, on with the show.

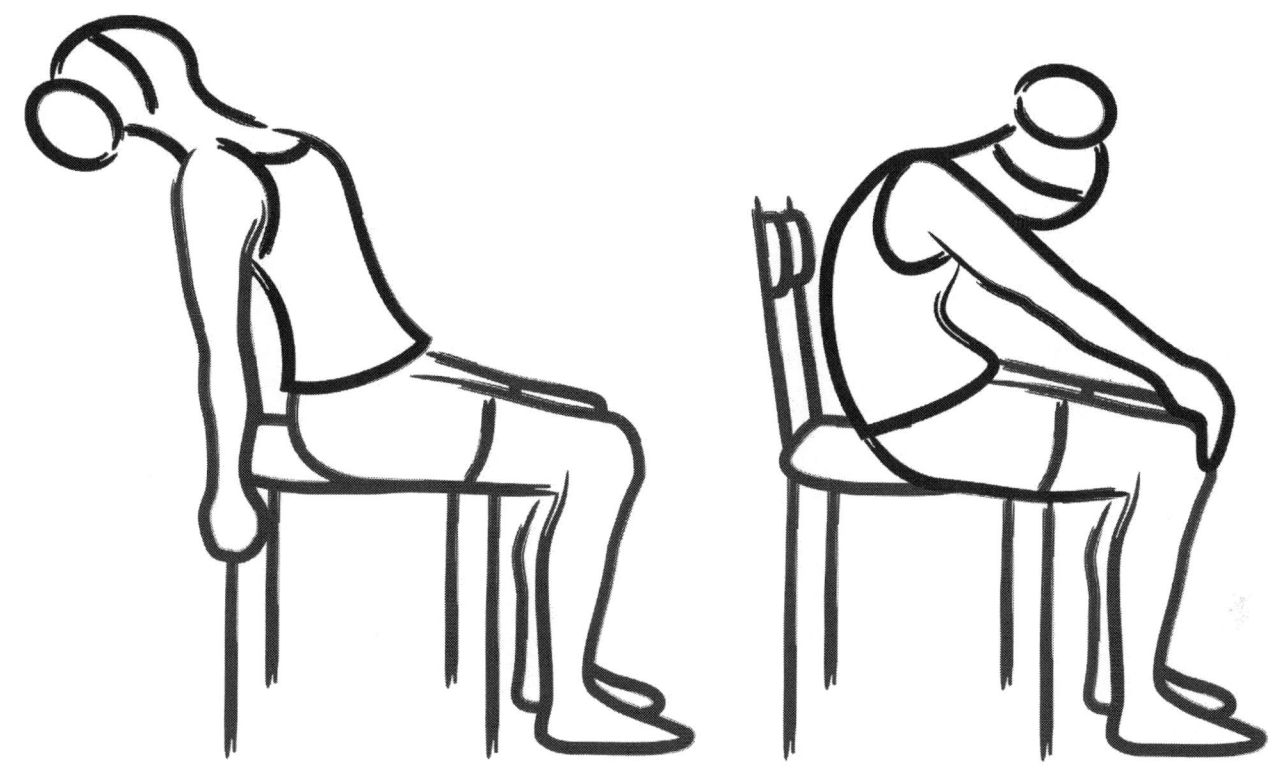

Seated Cat-Cow Stretch

This is a modification of the traditional cat-cow stretch usually practiced on the floor, helping to stretch and relieve the back and activate the core. To get into cat-cow stretch in a chair:

- Sit on your chair, planting your feet flat on the floor. Rest the hands on your knees and your thighs.
- Breathe in, arch the back, and shift your gaze to the ceiling to assume the cow pose. You should feel the stretch along the lower back.

- Breathe out and round the back, bringing the chin toward the chest to assume the cat pose. Feel the stretch along the upper back and activate in the core.
- Repeat this for 8 to 10 reps, stretching as far as is comfortable in each direction.

This movement is perfect for mobilizing your spinal flexion and extension right through your upper and lower back. The aim is to feel a strong but comfortable and controlled stretch in both the cat and cow position.

Once you feel confident with the cat-cow motion, try to activate your core muscles each time you return from the stretched positions to your neutral (sitting upright) position by drawing your belly button in towards the spine a little as you move.

Notes:

Sometimes, if your thoracic spine (upper back) is a little restricted or generally stiff, you may have a few clicking sounds as your spine starts to learn how to lengthen.

I have had clients panic a little in the past, which is understandable. As a general rule of thumb here, if you're smoothly controlling the movement without forcing it, and it clicks a few times while remaining pain-free, it's not a problem. It's most likely your spine finding range of movement that it hasn't been able to access for a while. Think of it like the clicks you might hear your back make if you visited a chiropractor.

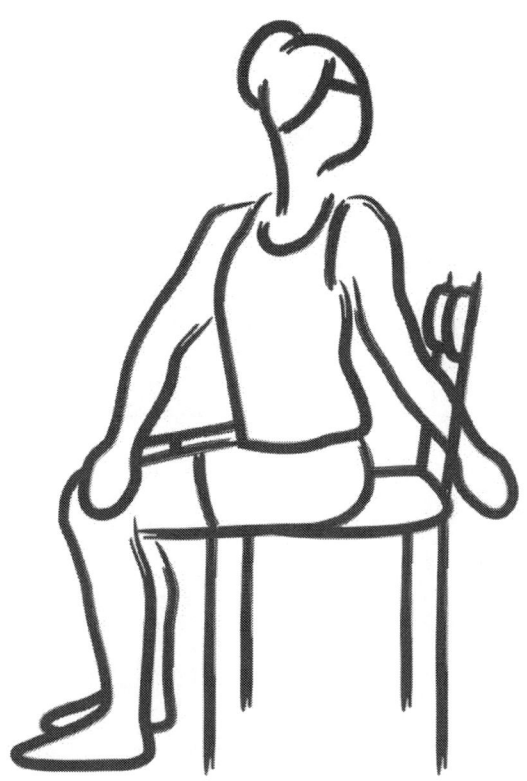

Seated Spinal Twist

Seated Spinal Twists help stretch out the spine and open up the muscles on both sides. Focus on pushing yourself enough to feel a nice stretch along the side you twist to. You can even reach out and feel that nice stretch as you go. To get into a seated spinal twist:

- Sit up tall and plant your feet on the floor.
- Rest your right hand on the outside of the left thigh and place the left hand behind the chair.
- Breathe in and out. As you breathe out, twist to your left until you feel a stretch, even if it is just a little bit here.

- Hold the position for 20 to 30 seconds, feeling the stretch and releasing the tension on that side.
- Release and repeat on the opposite side.

When you first try the seated spinal twist, you may not be able to rotate your body very far. Your goal as you improve is for you to be able to rotate your body to the point that you can comfortably look over your shoulder and see behind you.

If you're not quite there yet and only have the range to twist far enough to comfortably see to the side, but you can feel the stretch in the right place, then you are doing a fantastic job. Feeling the stretch in the right place is more important than your starting range of movement.

Don't think of any of the poses and movements that we work on together as a race to get to maximum range. By consistently practicing your chair yoga, you will gain the flexibility, mobility, and stability that you need to increase your controllable range of movement. So, keep that in mind as you practice, and keep up the good work.

YOUR FIRST CHAIR YOGA POSES

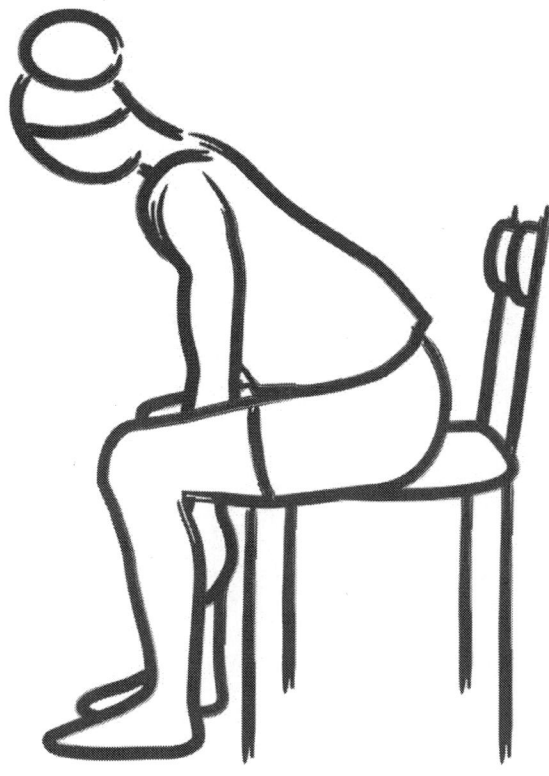

Seated Forward Folds

In the seated forward folds pose, you will need to sit on the edge of your seat, so pick a chair that can support that movement. This one is great for working on the core and the back, bringing the body up and down like a hinge. To get into seated forward folds:

- Sit on the edge of the chair and plant your feet hip-width apart on the floor. Sit comfortably.
- When you are ready, take a breath in and sit up straight. As you breathe out, hinge at the hips and fold your body forward.

- Slide your hands down the inside or front of your shins. If you don't feel ready to hinge your body that far at the moment, rest your hands on your thighs instead, whichever feels the most comfortable.
- Hold this position for 20 to 30 seconds. Active your core muscles by gently drawing your abs in and the return to your sitting upright position.

The aim when returning to your starting position is to use your core strength and glutes to move your body fully hinged (flexed forwards) to sitting upright. If your core needs a little assistance to begin with, place your hands on your thighs and push upward with your arms. As you gain strength (in your core, glutes, and back) through range, you will need your arms to push you up less and less.

This movement is, of course, a nice back stretch, but it's also so much more. It strengthens your body's ability to lift itself from a fully bent-over position into an upright posture. This action translates into so many real-life scenarios, making it incredibly important to maintain an active lifestyle. Examples of this include lifting something heavy from the floor, getting something out of the oven, or even climbing down into a swimming pool when you're on your next holiday! Without laboring my point much more, from this chapter, one of the key points I would like you to take away is the importance that your core muscles and spinal range play in keeping your body fit, healthy, and pain-free.

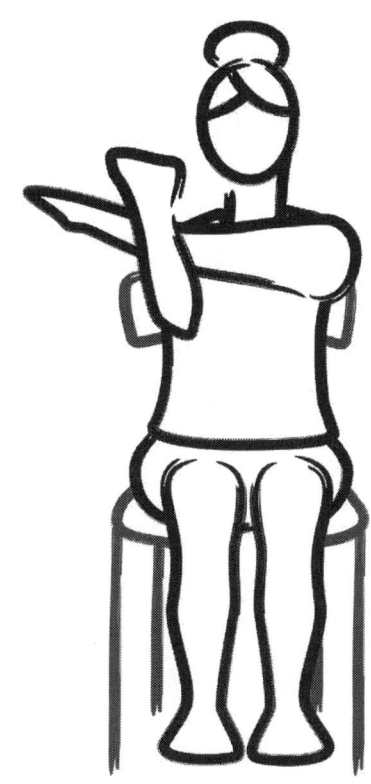

Seated Shoulder Stretch

While many chair yoga poses will focus on the back and core muscles, this one will focus on building range in your shoulders. You need those shoulders in good working order for lifting, reaching, and carrying through life. To get into a seated shoulder stretch:

- Sit on your chair, using the back as support if needed. Plant your feet flat on the ground.
- Take the left arm and lift it straight ahead of you, stopping at shoulder height.
- Take your left arm across your center line towards your right shoulder, keeping it long (outstretched) but loose at the elbow.

- Press your right hand against the back of the left upper arm to form a little resistance and increase the stretch.
- Hold this position for 15 to 30 seconds and bring the arms down for a break.
- Repeat the steps above on your other side, and complete 3 sets on each arm.

As you advance, try not to take a rest between switching sides. Also, to increase the intensity, try holding the stretch position for longer (45 seconds +) and give the stretches a little extra resistance.

Note:

Some important notes that apply to all stretches are:

- Always move smoothly in and out of a stretch so you can better control its intensity.
- Never rush into a stretched position or pose.
- Develop your flexibility by practicing consistently rather than trying to achieve maximum range in a day.

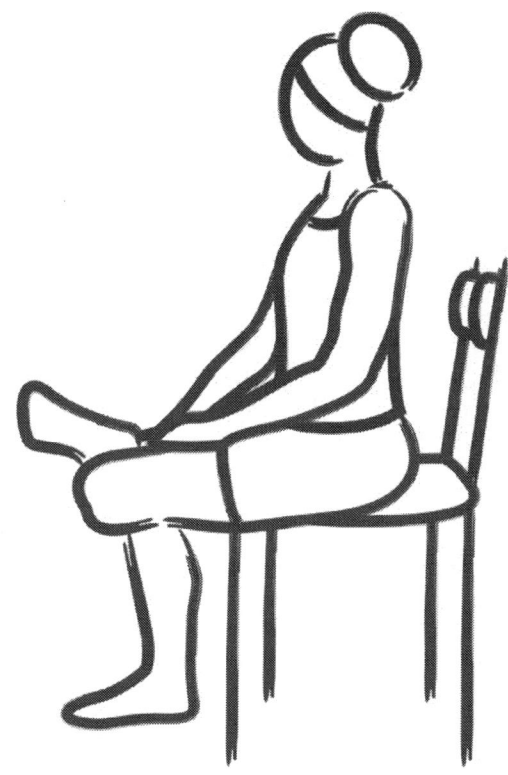

Seated Ankle-to-Knee Stretch

Hip health is incredibly important but often overlooked until there's a problem. Your hips are thought of as the powerhouse of the body. They are responsible for:

- Any squatting action you make, such as sitting down and standing back up again.
- Supporting and propel us forward as we walk or run.
- Protecting our lower backs and knees from soreness and injury.
- Alongside your core muscles, they hold you upright and are constantly reacting to correct your balance, preventing you from falling.

All of this without you needing to think about it!

The seated ankle-to-knee stretch helps you to build usable range in your hips to keep that remarkable machine that is your body working as it should, without any unnecessary resistance due to reduced range.

To get into a seated ankle-to-knee stretch:

- Sit in your chair and plant your feet flat on the ground.
- Rest your left ankle across your right knee.
- Flare your left knee out to the side, allowing it to pivot on your right leg and hang. Breathe in. As you breathe out and relax your body, let gravity do its work, and your left knee will gently lower itself creating a deep stretch in your left hip and glute (by the way, your glutes are the main muscles that make up your butt).
- Hold this pose for 30 to 45 seconds before releasing the stretch and repeating it on the other side.

As your range increases and you're ready for a deeper stretch, simply push down on your thigh on the side that you're stretching. This downward force pivots your hip further, increasing its lateral rotation and intensifying the stretch. If you're trying this out, apply the downward force slowly and smoothly, as with all stretches; the intensity will jump from 0 to 60 very quickly.

YOUR FIRST CHAIR YOGA POSES

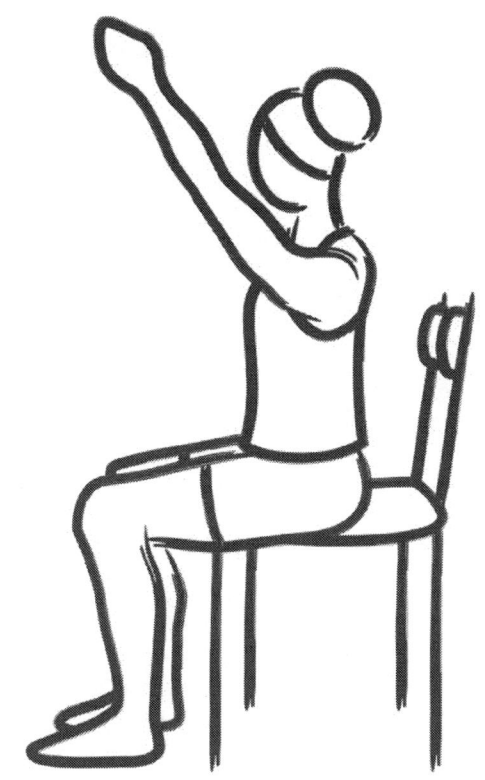

Seated Urdhva Hastasana

The focus of this pose is to build range in your shoulder joints while using your arms as a downward driver to load and unload your upper back. This means that as you raise and lower your arms, their movement applies a downward force on your upper back, and to maintain your posture, you must brace your body against it.

Even though it's a simple up-and-down arm movement, I would like you to focus on maintaining an upright seated posture and to activate your core muscles by drawing in your abs as you practice it.

To get into this position:

- Sit upright on the chair. Ideally, slightly away from the backrest so that you have to use your postural muscles and core strength. If you feel that you are unable to do this to begin with, slide back in your chair and start out using the backrest until you are confident with your form.
- On the inhale, raise your arms towards the ceiling while drawing your shoulder blades together and downwards. Imagine that you have an invisible pencil that you're trying to gently grip between your shoulder blades as you move. If you feel stiff and can't raise the arms all the way up, then just go as high as you can.
- Hold the arms there for a count of 20 seconds and take several controlled breaths in and out while maintaining your posture and drawing in your abs.
- Slowly lower your arms until they are at your sides. Repeat for 5 to 10 repetitions.

If you find that you are unable to maintain your posture while reaching high overhead, reduce your reach on the next repetition, as without wanting to sound like a broken record; form comes first!

While your arms are in the air, try to extend your thoracic spine (upper spine) as much as you can. This will help you to build your mind/muscle connection between your posture, your shoulders, and your core.

To begin with, if your range is restricting your ability to maintain an upright posture throughout the movement, just reduce your range, even if that means that you start with your arms only slightly elevated. By adapting the pose to work with how you move, you'll build your strength and range much faster than if you force the movement.

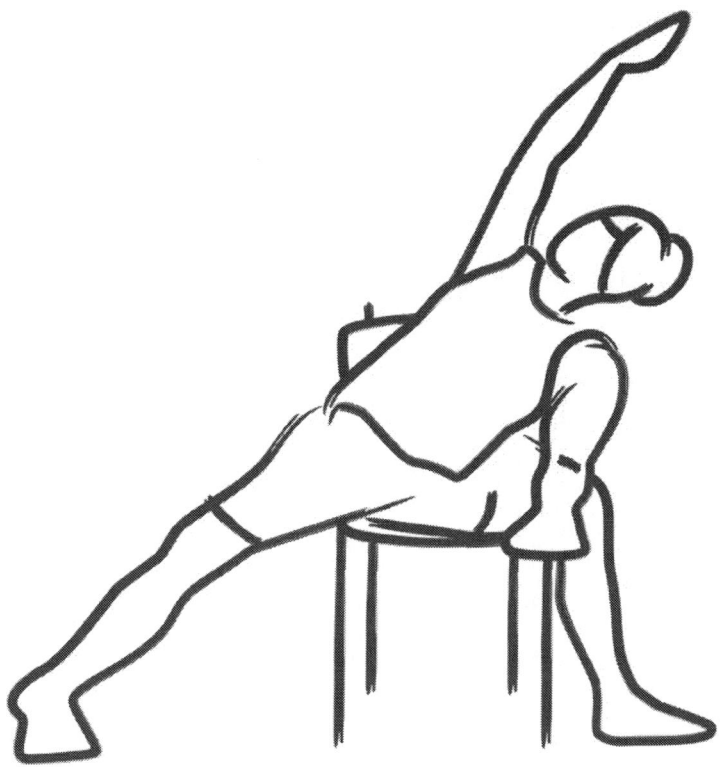

Chair Extended Side Angle

Aside from being a great stretch that lengthens the sides of your body out when held, the chair extended side angle also opens and builds the range in your hips, builds strength and stability in your ankles, knees, and thighs, mobilizes your shoulder range, and is even said to help improve digestion!

This is one of the high-skill poses where chair yoga really comes into its own. As you can probably imagine, as a beginner (or even at an intermediate level), holding this pose and maintaining good form without the support of a chair would be extremely difficult. By using the chair, you can practice your form safely while still gaining all the benefits.

To get into the chair extended side angle:

- Start by sitting in an upright position in your chair, and once again, activate your core muscles by drawing your abs in.
- Keeping your left knee flexed at 90 degrees, rotate your hips to the left, and face your left foot out to the side. Notice how the back of your thigh (your hamstrings) on your left leg are now on the chair's seat and taking your weight.
- Hinge your hips, fold your body forward towards your left knee, and lean your left arm on top of your left thigh for support.
- Once you feel supported, extend your right leg out to the opposite side until it's completely straight. Glace back and adjust the foot on your straight leg so that it is flat on the floor and facing forward. Something to be aware of: even though your outstretched leg is straight, try not to lock out your knee.
- Now that your legs are in the correct position, let's focus on your upper body. While leaning on your left thigh with your left arm, take a deep inhale. Now rotate your body to the right, extend your right arm overhead to expand your chest, and complete the pose. As you reach overhead with your right arm, exhale.
- Breathe slowly and deeply while you hold the position. Count 5 to 10 breaths before lowering your right arm and returning to your start position before repeating on the other side.

If you would like to push yourself a little further in this pose, try straightening your supporting arm (your left arm in the example teaching points) and reach it down the outside of your thigh until your fingertips touch the floor. This is a tough challenge, but with a little practice, you'll be able to do it.

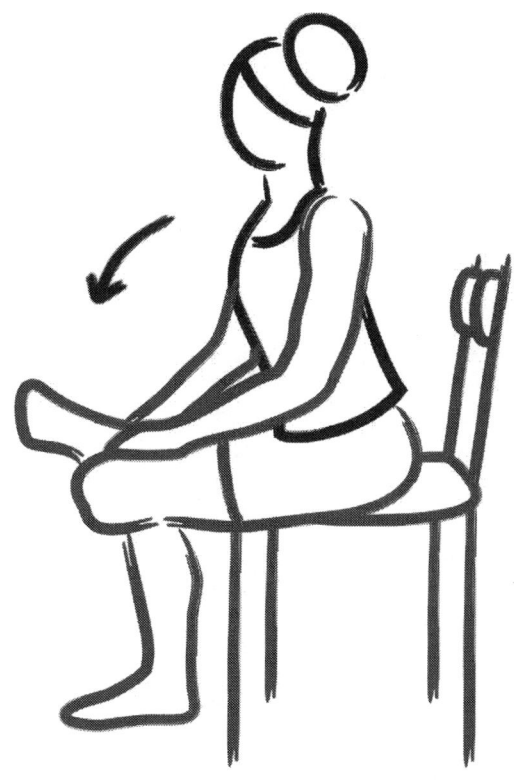

Chair Pigeon

Similar to the seated ankle-to-knee stretch, the chair pigeon pose will help you to open up your hip range and glute flexibility. The main difference is that the intensity of the stretch is controlled by how far you hinge your hips and tip your body forward.

To get into Chair Pigeon:

- Sit up straight, focusing on good posture to start.
- Follow the teaching points for the ankle-to-knee stretch.
- Now that you're in an ankle-to-knee stretch hinge your hips, tip your body forward, lowering your chest toward your legs. Hold this position for 5 to 10 breaths before releasing. Repeat the stretch 2 more times before switching to the other side.

Building range, strength, and stability in your hips teaches your body to use them more effectively when you move, which will de-load your lower back and your knees in the process. I have helped so many clients greatly reduce or totally eradicate lower back pain, both as a one-to-one coach and as a sports therapist, simply by improving their hip functionality.

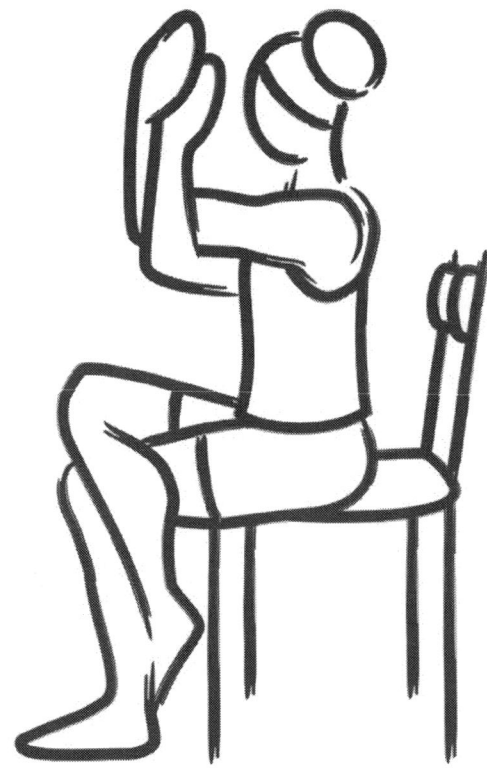

Chair Eagle

Okay, I know what you're thinking. This pose looks like a crazy tangle, so how on Earth will it actually benefit me?

To put it simply, the chair eagle improves muscle tone, circulation, and flexibility. Not bad for a crazy tangle! It also builds strength and range in your hips, ankles, fingers, wrists, and elbows while simultaneously reducing stiffness in your neck and shoulders.

At first, you may want to start working on getting your leg position right before adding the arms in for the full pose. The aim is to feel the stretch in your thighs and shoulders as you wind your arms and legs around each other. Remember to activate your core muscles, as we've been practicing in your previous poses, to keep you stable on your chair. To get into a chair eagle pose:

- Sit in an upright position on your chair and then cross your right thigh over the left.
- The aim is to wrap your right foot all the way around the back of your left calf. If you don't quite have the flexibility yet, then just take it to a level where you can feel your thigh muscles brace, and you can hold the position comfortably under tension.
- Next, cross your left arm over your right, meeting at the elbows. Bend both elbows and touch your palms together. If you don't quite have the range to touch your palms together yet, then take it to a level where you can hold the position under tension, just like we talked about with your chair eagle leg position.
- Now that your legs and arms are in position, slowly and smoothly lift your elbows up to, or as near as you can comfortably get, to chest height, and draw your shoulders back and down at the same time, making your neck feel long and straight. Hold position for 5 slow, deep breaths before releasing. Take a moment and repeat on the other side.

If you find it tough to get into this pose, all that it means is that your body probably needs it!

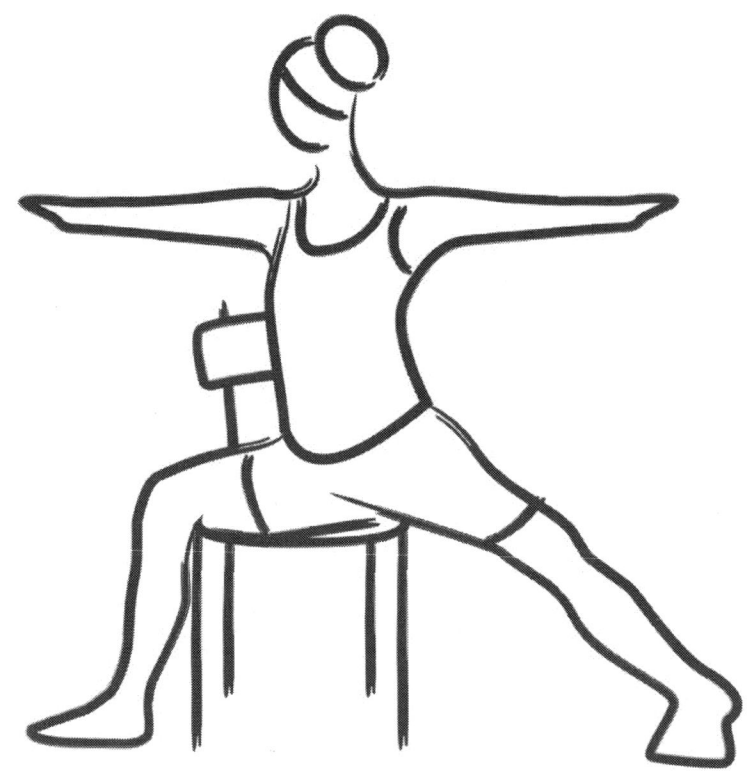

Chair Warrior II

Now we are getting down to some of the poses that you are more likely to recognize. Warrior II is a great stretch for both the upper and lower body. It opens your chest and shoulders while also building strength, range, and stability in your hips and legs. As you can probably imagine, holding this pose without the support of a chair is tough at first, but it's something that I know you will be able to accomplish as your balance, strength, and coordination improve. Until then, let's stick with the chair version so that you can practice safely and build your body and skill level with confidence.

Try the following teaching points below for the Chair Warrior II pose:

- Start in a sitting upright position.
- Now follow the steps to position your lower body as we walked through previously for the seated side angle pose. For this description, have your right knee at 90 degrees and your left leg outstretched straight.
- Focus on rooting your feet to the floor, lengthening your back and posture, and activating your core muscles.
- Now, take a deep breath in. As you exhale, extend your arms to your sides, palms down, and raise them up to shoulder height. Focus on drawing your shoulder blades back and down, feeling your chest open into a comfortable stretch.
- Try to line up your arms so that they are directly over your legs while keeping your body upright, your leg muscles braced, and your feet rooted.
- Make your neck as long as comfortably possible (I like to imagine a piece of string attached to my crown being gently pulled directly upward for this). Now gently draw your chin back and in while looking over the fingertips of your outstretched right arm.
- Hold the position for 5 controlled breaths before lowering your arms and returning to a sitting upright position.
- Repeat on the other side up to three sets per side. I also recommend that you alternate sides between sets. This will help to

improve your dynamic hip range and your ability to get in and out of the pose.

Note:

Always remember that good form is paramount. If that means, that to begin with, you feel like you're not going that deep into the stretch or can only manage one set, that's totally fine. Over the coming weeks of practice, as your leg strength, hip range, and overall stability improve, so will all of your yoga poses.

I'd just like to make a quick side note to talk about the neck position described in these teaching points. I want you to think of it this way: your head sits on top of your spine, acting like a weight at the end of a chain. The position of your head acts as a downward driver (remember how we described upward and downward drivers earlier) on your spine, so as it leans forward, your spine pushes backward to compensate.

By positioning your head as described in the chair warrior II teaching points while elongating your spine, helps to build range in your thoracic spine (upper spine), particularly where many people have formed what's known as a kyphosis (dowager's hump in layman's terms) due to constant flexion.

The key to building range is not to force it but instead to do it gradually and allow your body to adapt to the new movements and overloads that you're putting upon it. I want you to take a moment to realize how well you're doing. You have already learned a lot, so big well done for sticking with it. Now, onto the final chair yoga pose for this chapter.

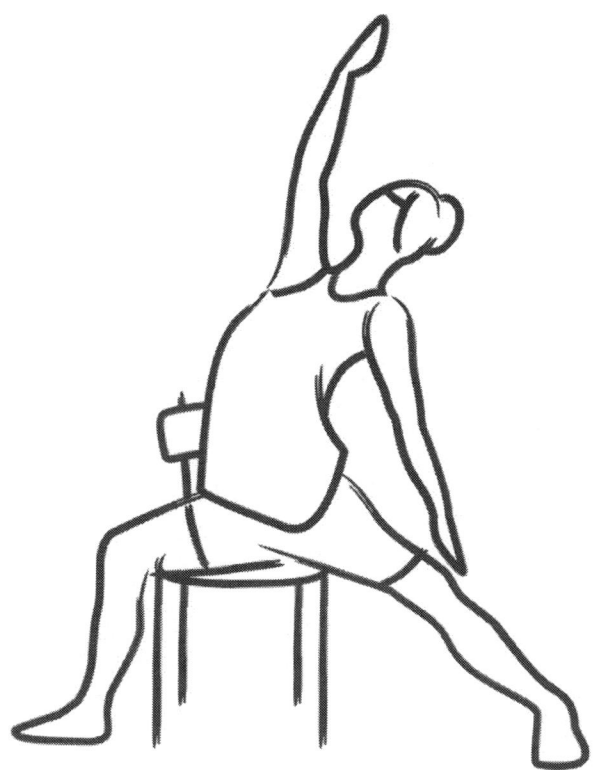

Reverse Chair Warrior

As you can probably tell, the reverse chair warrior is an adaptation of the chair warrior II pose. The focus here is to use your arms as a downward driver to further extend your spine and activate your core muscles under control. You're looking to access range in your hips and back that you may not have used in quite some time, so take your time and move with smooth control.

To get into the reverse chair warrior pose:

- Like always, start by sitting upright on your chair.

- Now get yourself into a full chair warrior II pose (right leg forward and at 90 degrees, left leg extended out straight).
- Once there, lower your left arm towards your left knee while simultaneously raising your right arm overhead (right palm facing behind you once overhead).
- Take a deep breath in. As you exhale, reach your right arm overhead and behind you, allowing it to act as a downward driver to extend your back. Use your left arm for support on your left leg if you need to.
- Hold this pose for 3 to 5 deep breaths before using your core muscles to pull you back to a relaxed chair warrior II position.
- Take 3 to 5 breaths before repeating for 5 repetitions.
- Once you have completed your set, switch sides and repeat.

I know that I say this a lot, but I'll say it again anyway. Listen to your body and be consistent!

If you're new to chair yoga and just getting started on a new fitness journey, it's okay to start out small and work to improve a little more each day. You'll be amazed by the results you can achieve in as little as 21 days just by being consistent and making small, incremental improvements each day. It's not about trying to master every pose in a week; it's about giving your body a chance to adapt to the new overloads that you're placing on it while strengthening that all-important mind/muscle connection.

You'll notice that now I have really dug into the movements, such as what are and how to use upward and downward drivers, how to activate your core muscles, and so on, that my teaching points will become sorter and sharper as I don't want to over labor the points. That being said, at a later stage in the book, if you can't remember what something means and need to refresh your memory, please refer back to this chapter, and hopefully it'll put you back on the right path.

We've already learned so much together, and I'm excited for us to move on to the next chapter.

FREE BONUS:
CHAIR YOGA POSES EXERCISES CHART

As I mentioned previously, to prevent you from having to prop up this book while practicing your chair yoga poses, I have put together each of the exercises pictured in this chapter into a video guide and an enlarged and printable chart to make it easier to follow. To get your free chair yoga pose charts, head to bit.ly/chair-yoga-free in your internet browser, and I email over your copy.

You can also scan the QR Code below with your cell phone camera and tap on the link that pops up if you find that easier.

I hope that you find it helpful.

3

STANDING AND FLOOR BASED YOGA POSES *(WITH CHAIR MODIFICATIONS)*

"Success is the sum of small efforts, repeated day in and day out."

- ROBERT COLLIER

As you progress through your yoga routines over the coming weeks, you will feel your body gaining strength and becoming more flexible, and you will notice how much steadier you feel in general. When I'm coaching a client one-to-one, one of the things that I love most is watching how quickly their self-confidence grows as they get into the swing of their daily practice and as they see the results they have earned.

As you feel yourself becoming stronger, you can progress your poses and eventually remove the chair altogether. There is such a variety of exercises and poses that yoga has to offer that I hope that once you perfect the seated poses, you at least consider trying some of the chairless alternatives. With that in mind, allow me to show you some standing and lying down yoga poses for you to practice when you are ready. If you don't feel ready yet, that's no problem at all. Just skip over this chapter and come back to it at a later date.

Standing Yoga Poses

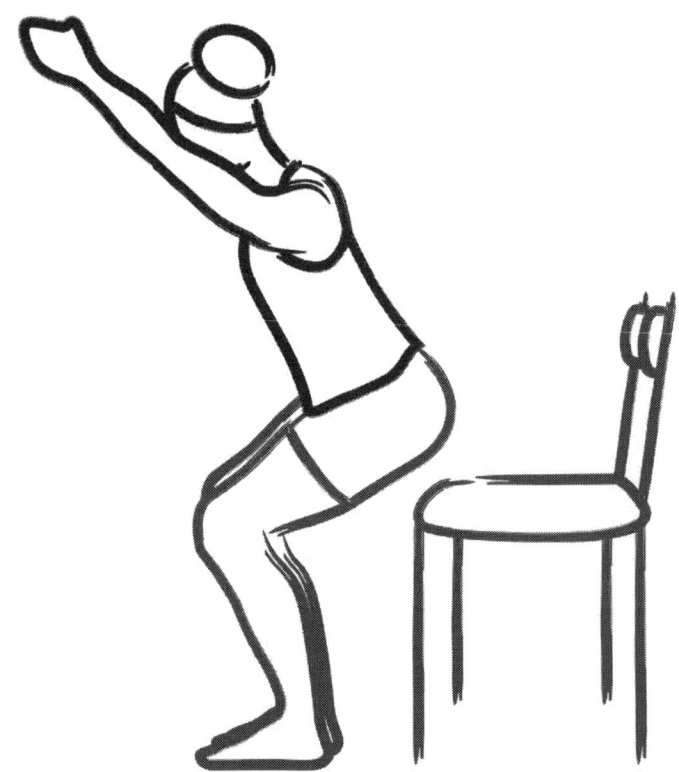

Chair Pose

The main purpose of the chair pose is to strengthen your thighs and stabilize your knees. How strong your legs are and how stable you are underfoot is a cornerstone of an independent and active life, making the chair pose a real winner. Even though this pose is simple, that does not make it easy! To get into the chair pose:

- Stand in front of your chair with your feet together or hips distance apart. Extend the arms directly over your head, drawing your shoulder blades back and down.
- Take a breath in. As you exhale, slowly sit towards your chair, hinging your hips back and bending your knees while keeping your feet flat on the floor. Go down as far as you can, with the ultimate goal of getting your thighs parallel to the ground so that you're hovering just above your chair's seat.
- Try to breathe normally and hold the pose for 30 to 60 seconds before driving back up to a standing position.

Your goal with this pose is to squat and hold as low as a chair with a strong upright posture. The key here is in the holding of the position rather than how deep you can go. Only squat down to a range that you can hold position. Once you can hold for longer than 30 seconds, try increasing the depth of your chair pose to add intensity.

If you're finding this pose too difficult to hold, try it with your back against a wall to give you something to brace against and reduce the difficulty.

Note:

There are some bonus points I would like you to think about. When entering a squat position, always make sure that your knees align with your toes. The body often wants our knees to fall inward as we squat, which is a big no-no while exercising. When your knees fall inward, they cause unequal loading of the muscles, signaling your glutes to switch off, and it is also highly likely to increase wear and tear on your knees.

Something else that is worth mentioning here is that there are three main types of muscle contraction: as you lift (concentric), as you release (eccentric), and when you brace and hold (isometric). In the case of the chair pose, you are using an isometric contraction effectively to hold you steady and build stability in your knees and legs. Anyway, on with the yoga.

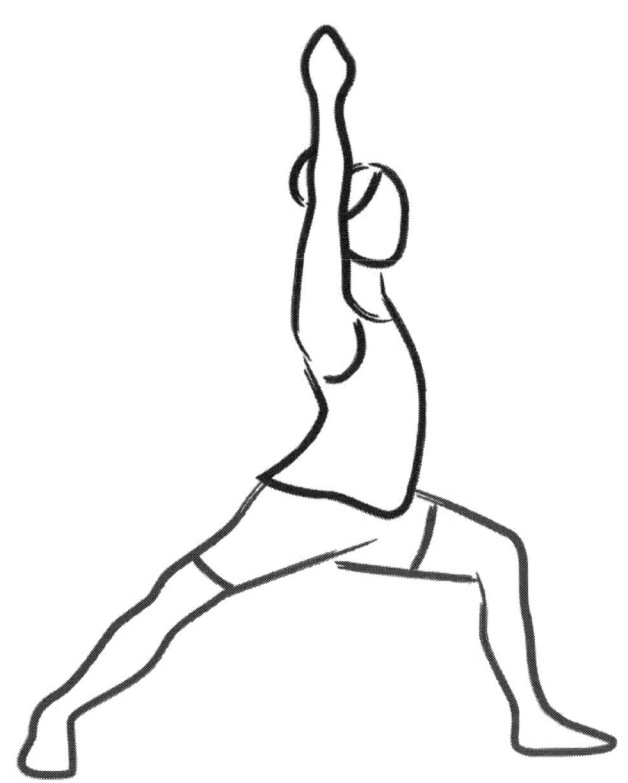

Warrior 1

Warrior poses mainly target and strengthen the quads, hamstrings, and core muscles. You can choose your level of intensity based on your current flexibility and skill level. To get into the warrior 1 pose:

- Stand with your feet together and keep the arms loose by your sides.
- Step forward with the left foot out into a lunge. The right leg (rear leg) should be straight with the foot at a 45-degree angle.
- Extend your arms overhead, gently squeezing your shoulder blades together and down. Move the head to look up at your fingers or straight ahead.
- Hold the pose for 30 seconds before releasing. Repeat on the other side.

At first, your lunge may be shallow as you work to improve your balance and strength. As your legs get stronger, and similar to the chair pose, push yourself and test your hold depth to increase the intensity.

Even though it's fairly obvious, and seeing as we've already practiced the warrior II and the reverse warrior poses on a chair in the previous chapter, I wanted to show you the chair equivalent for the chair warrior I. While you get to grips with the position, and if you would like the chance to test your range and build confidence in the pose itself, perhaps attempt the chair warrior 1 before the full warrior 1. I leave this up to you to decide.

To get into the chair warrior 1 pose:

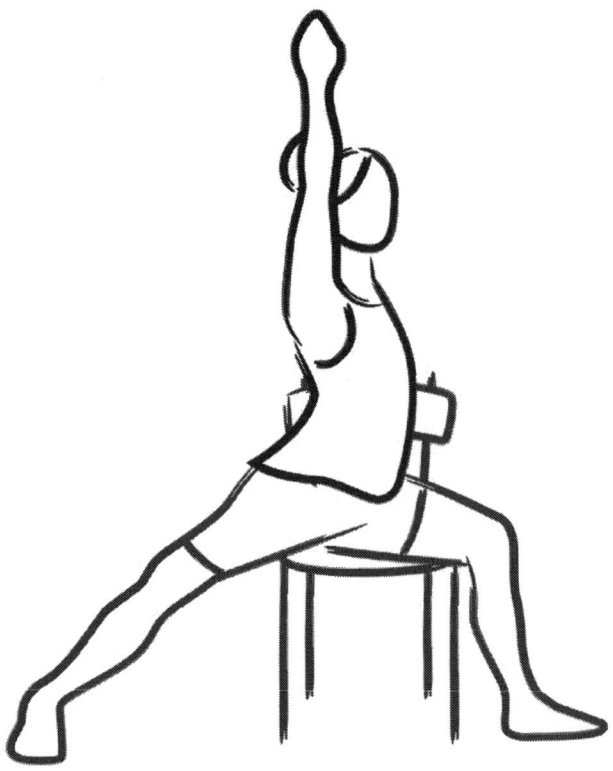

- Face forward and take the left leg out to the side of the chair at a right angle.
- Turn the rest of the body so you face to the left, in the same direction as your leg is going.
- Stretch out the right leg all the way, letting the toes touch the ground behind you. You should feel a stretch similar to being in a lunge but remain sitting.
- When you feel the stretch and can maintain balance, stretch the arms above the head. Hold for 30 counts before releasing and repeating on the other side.

It is okay if you need to start practicing this pose in a seated position if you feel this will help you to really nail the form. As I've mentioned several times already, form is always first!

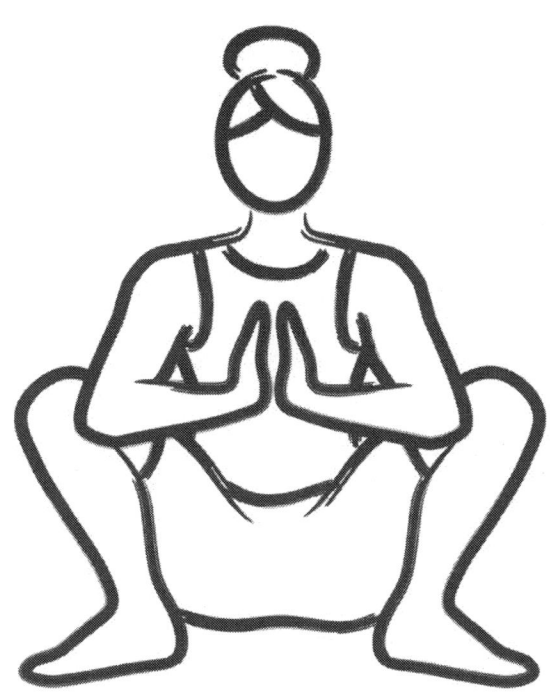

The Garland

The Garland pose helps to tone your core, aids digestion, and supports overall hip health, which makes it a brilliant addition to your yoga routine. Try not to be put off if you think it looks too difficult for you at this stage; I have included two more variations using a chair to ensure that anybody at any level will still be able to gain this pose's awesome benefits.

From a fitness perspective, the aim of the Garland pose is to build strength, stability, and mobility in your entire lower body while also developing your mind/muscle connection between your leg muscles and your core.

The good thing about the Garland pose is that it offers therapeutic and relaxation benefits as well. It helps to release and relax your hips and lower back while also stretching your inner thigh muscles.

Your goal for the end of today is to try versions of this pose (whether that's using a chair or free-standing) so that you can feel the benefits for yourself.

To perform a free-standing Garland pose:

- Stand up straight, keeping the feet as close together as possible. Let the toes point out.
- Start to squat down. Let the torso fall between your thighs, pressing the elbows against the knees.
- Make sure your tailbone is pressed to the ground and your chest is up. The resistance in your knees should help.
- Hold the position for 30 to 60 seconds.

One of the beauties of exercise is that it can and should be adapted to suit your current training. With that in mind, as promised above, here are some alternative versions of the Garland pose. Try one that you think will work for you.

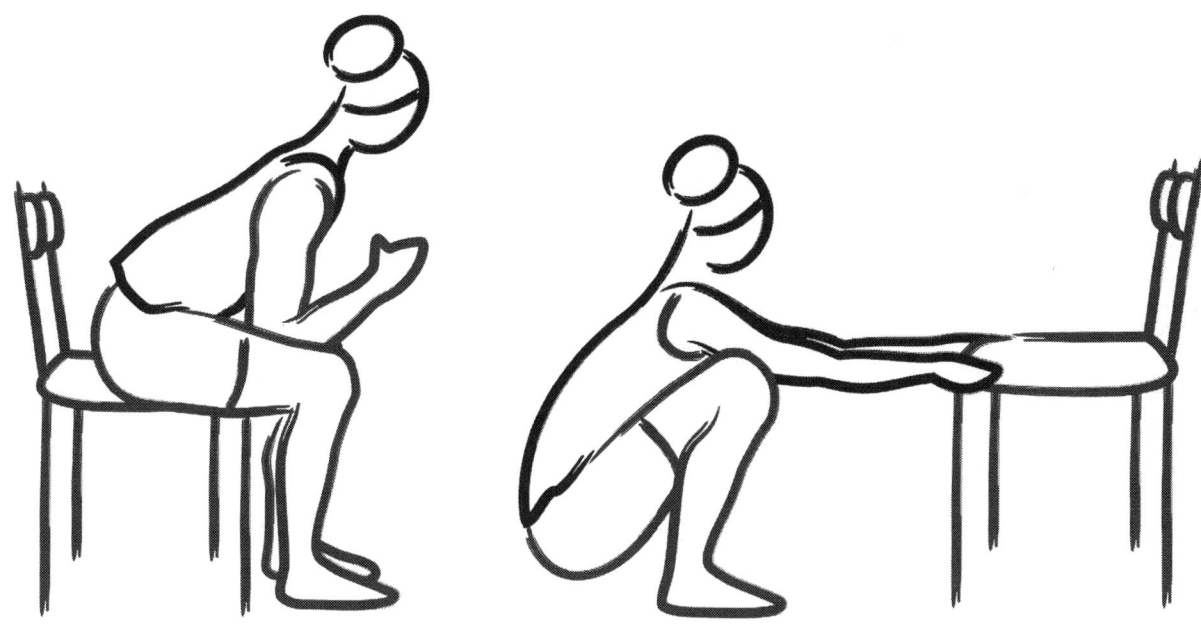

You can either sit on or hold onto your chair for support to help keep your balance and maintain the correct position. It's worth mentioning that if you're holding onto the chair for balance like in the image in the above right image, don't lean backward and hang against it as the chair might move or topple. In both of the chair variations, follow the teaching points for the free-standing Garland pose while incorporating your chair as shown. Remember to stay focused on what you should be feeling. Progress at your own rate and enjoy your results.

Note:

The goal is to gradually build your controllable strength through range. If your movement feels restricted at first or you feel unstable if you push the depth to begin with, that's fine. Your focus, as always, should be on maintaining good form. By maintaining good form, you will build your strength, balance, and range of motion quickly. Progress at your own rate.

Floor-Based Yoga Poses

When practicing any floor-based yoga positions, it's worth first making sure that you:

- Apart from your chair that can be used to help you to and from the floor, have a clear space all around you to avoid accidents.
- Use a yoga mat or comfortable flat surface to practice on.
- Use a cushion under your knees whenever your knees are in contact with the ground.

Following the above guidelines will help to keep your exercise comfortable and safe.

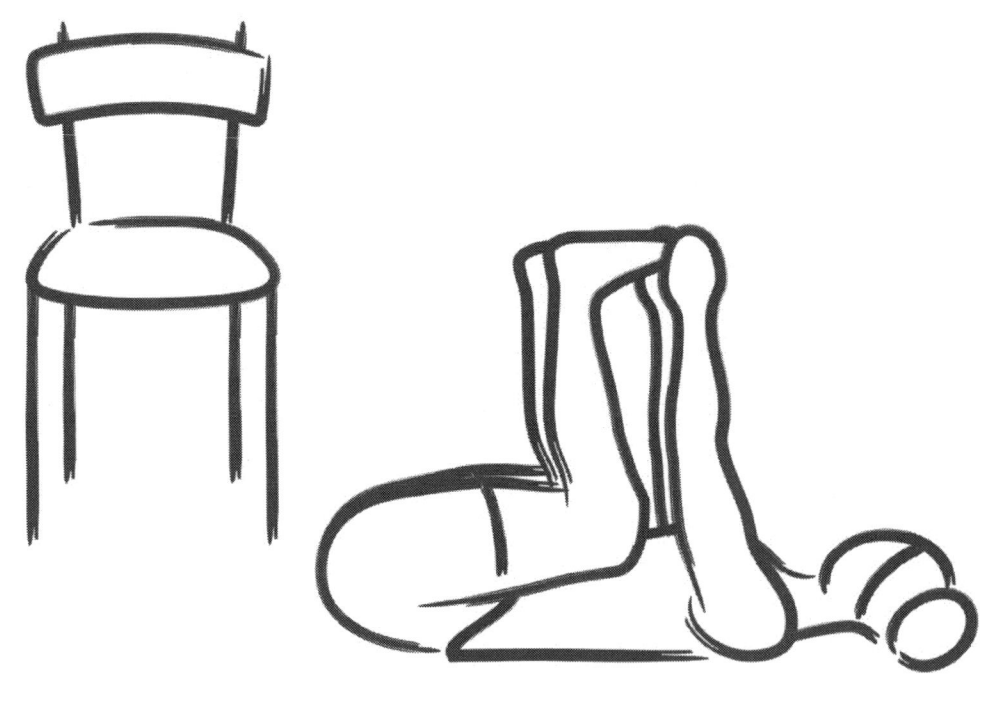

Happy Baby

Happy Baby may sound a little silly, but it is a brilliant stretch for the inner thighs, hips, and lower back. It has also been shown to reduce lower back pain, realign the spine, ease stress and anxiety, and lower your heart rate.

I have also included a chair variation of this pose, so you have the option.

To get into the happy baby pose:

- Lie down on the ground with your back flat.
- Bend your knees and inhale as you draw them up towards your chest, allowing them to slightly flare outward as you do. Grip the outsides of your feet with your hands.
- Keep your head and back on the floor and draw your chin towards your chest.
- Slowly exhale. As you exhale, press your tailbone into the floor as you gently push your feet upward against your hands to create tension.
- Now relax the tension and take another breath in.
- Repeat for 4 to 8 slow, controlled breaths.

If your range doesn't currently allow you to quite reach your feet yet, for now, grab onto the backs of your thighs instead.

Every time you practice the pose, you'll gain the benefits, and your range will develop until grabbing your feet will be no problem. Remember that we're looking for step-by-step progress, which happens through consistency over weeks rather than just going as hard as possible once.

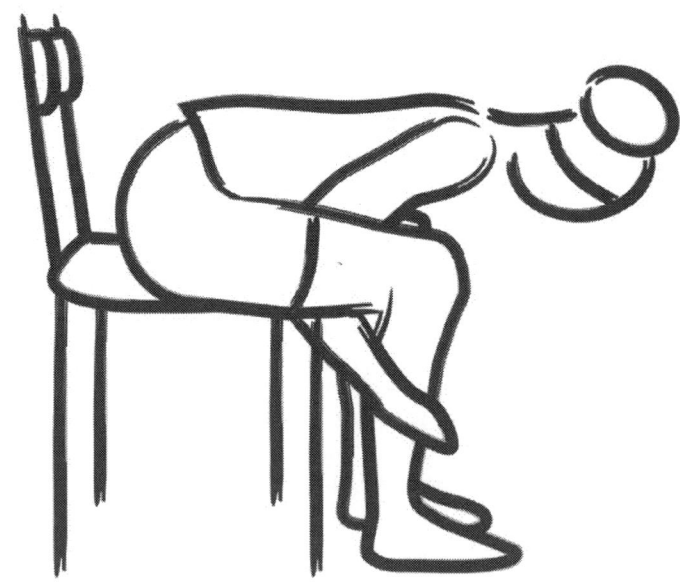

If you don't feel quite ready for the lying-down version of this pose just yet, there's a great version that you can work on while you are sitting in a chair (as shown above).

Start by folding your body forward, and then aim to hold (or touch with fingertips) just behind your knees. As your mobility and flexibility improve, and you can hinge your hips further, you can gradually reach further down your legs on each side to increase the intensity of the stretch.

STANDING AND FLOOR BASED YOGA POSES

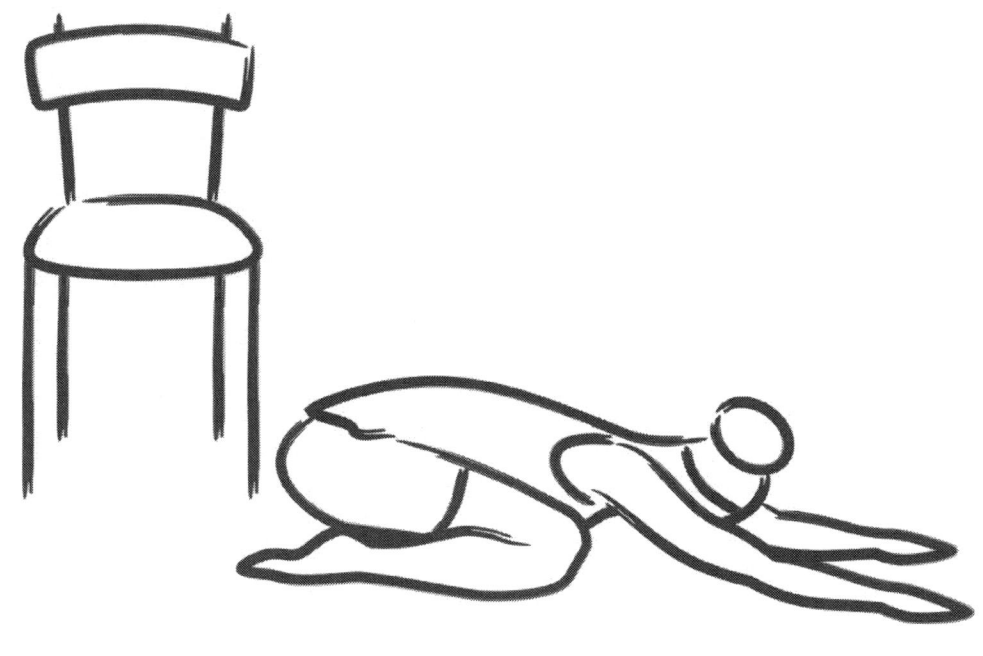

Child's Pose

Often described as a calming and grounding position, the child's pose has benefits for both your mind and body. Physically, it helps to lengthen your spine and open your hips and relieves tension in your back, neck, and pelvis. As this pose uses gravity rather than muscle tension to create range, as your body relaxes into position, it can help to quieten your mind and bring you to a state of mental calm.

To get into a child's pose:

- Start by getting down on all-fours. I recommend that you tuck a cushion under your knees, even if you're using a yoga mat, to help protect them and keep you comfortable.

- Flare your knees out to the sides, with your big toes to touching together behind you. This creates a space for your upper body to fold into. Now inhale.
- Hinge your body backward, allowing your stomach to fall between the thighs while bringing the forehead to the floor. Exhale as you move.
- Extend the arms in front of you, letting your palms rest on the floor. Once in position, breathe deeply, hinge backward, and allow your body to sink naturally.

Breathe deeply, bringing the chest as close to the floor as possible. Hold the stretch to releasing all the tension for a 30 to 60 seconds. You should feel a strong but comfortable stretch in your lower back and shoulders as you sink forward. You will also feel the stretch in your thighs and hips as you settle into the stretch.

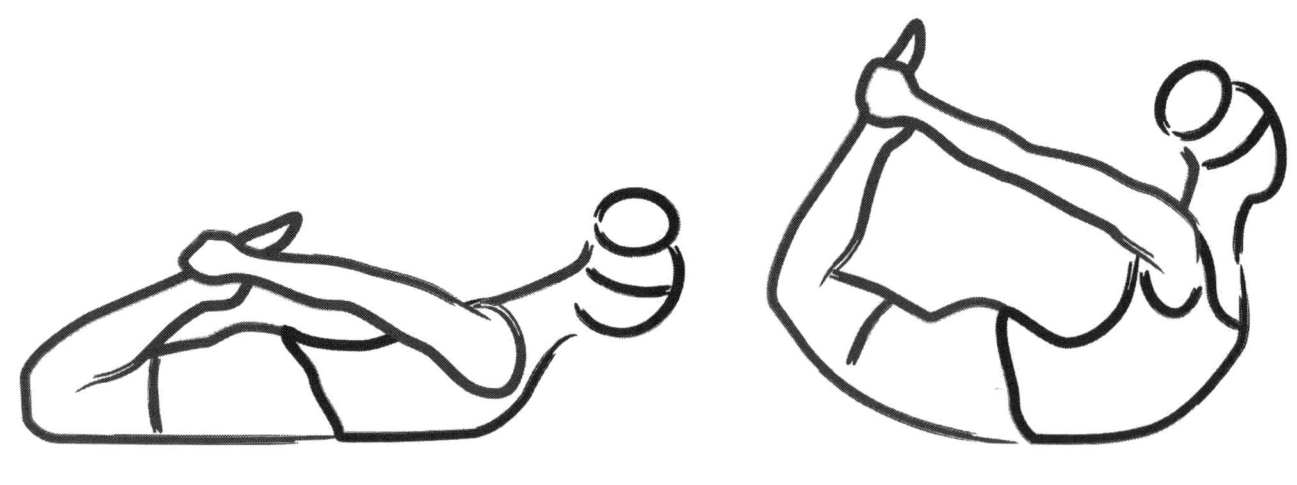

Bow

The bow pose is quite an advanced position. It helps to strengthen your postural muscles, including your neck and mid-back, while simultaneously releasing your chest and shoulders and building range through your whole spine. If you don't feel ready to try a full bow pose just yet don't worry, because I have also included a chair bow pose for you to start with so that you can still gain benefits as you work your way up to it.

To get into a full bow pose:

- Lie down on your stomach, with your arms to your sides, palms up.
- Bend your knees and reach back with your arms, grabbing your ankles with your hands and keeping the knees in line with the hips.
- As you take a deep breath in, gently pull your legs, lifting your thighs and your chest off the floor. Draw your shoulders back and look ahead. Brace your body and hold for up to 10 to 20 seconds before returning to the start position and relaxing.
- Repeat this for 5 to 10 repetitions. If you can, try adding a little more pain-free tension into it each time.

On your first attempt, if you manage one repetition or ten, that is amazing work. Big well done! This pose requires a good deal of core control and flexibility to accomplish. With practice, you will see rapid improvement.

I understand that you may be thinking, "Hold on a minute, I thought that this book was about Chair Yoga, so why are you showing me so many poses that don't use a chair?". There's a simple answer to this question: as your coach, I want to show you more than just the basics. I want to show you progressions that will take you from the level that you are at today and show you where it can take you if you stay focused and train consistently. All exercise programs should be progressive, and the best way to make continuous progress is to know the direction that you should be headed.

If you find the bow pose a little too challenging at the moment, then the chair equivalent is an excellent alternative.

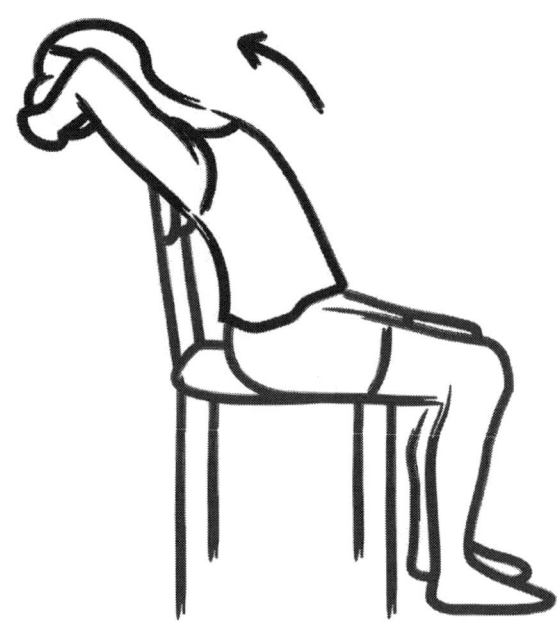

The main aim of the chair bow is to increase the range in your spine (including your neck) by extending it under control, using your head as a downward driver.

- Sit forward on your chair and plant your feet hip distance apart on the floor.
- Slowly lean back to find the chair's backrest with your upper back, cradle your head in your hands at the base of your skull (interlacing fingers works well), and flare your elbows out to the sides. Take a deep breath in.

STANDING AND FLOOR BASED YOGA POSES

- Now, use your chair's backrest as a pivot point, the weight of your head as a downward driver, and breathe out and extend your spine until you feel your whole body lengthen.
- Hold this pose for 10 to 20 seconds breathing normally before returning to an upright sitting position.
- Repeat for 5 to 10 repetitions.

Note:

When you lean back on your chair, you should make sure that you keep your hips and legs firm and braced downwards and slightly forwards as you extend your spine slowly to ensure that your chair doesn't tip backward. Remember that all movements are there to push your body for improvements, but they should always be pain-free.

On a side note, if the backrest on your chair feels as though it's too hard or is pressing into your back and making it sore as you pivot, I suggest that you hang a folded towel over it to make it feel more comfortable.

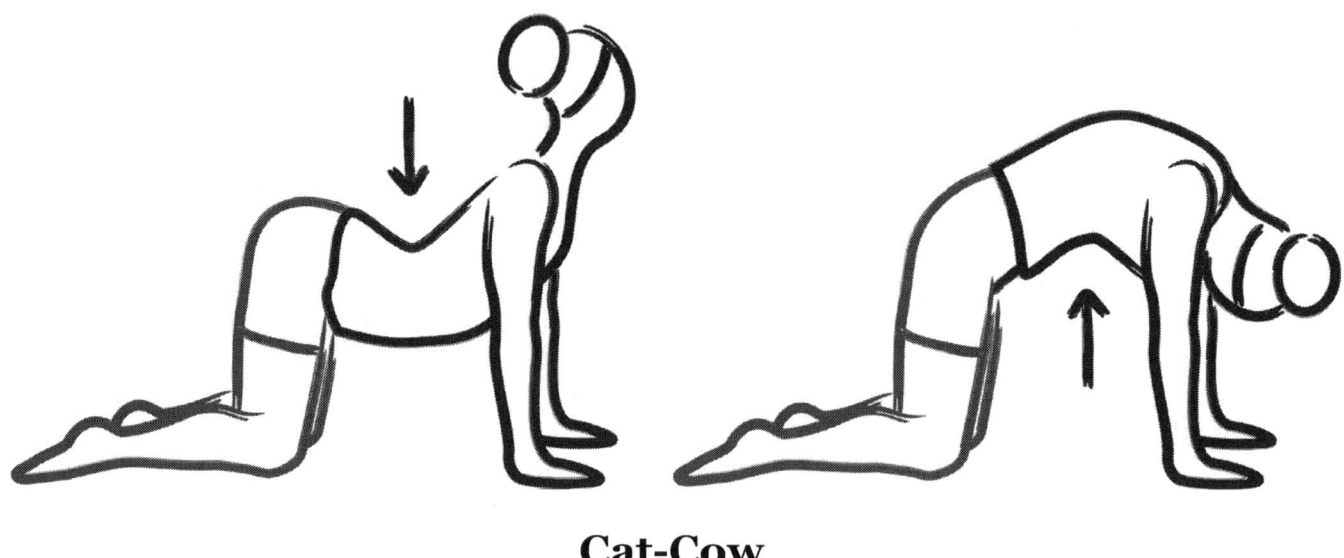

Cat-Cow

The cat-cow pose is an excellent way to bring dynamic mobility to the spine and neck by gently stretching your back while strengthening your core muscles and softly stimulating your abdominal organs. The aim of the movement is to gently flow from one position to the other in time with your breathing and to hold the peak of each movement for a count of 5 or 10 seconds. Animal noises are optional!

Here are the teaching points for the cat-cow:

- Get down onto all-fours on your mat, and place your hands under your shoulders and your knees under the hips. Any time you have to kneel down on the ground (even if you're on a mat), I often recommend that you tuck a cushion under your knees for comfort.
- Once in position, take a deep breath in. When ready, engage your core muscles and exhale while pushing your spine up toward the ceiling. As you do this, gently tuck your head and tailbone downward.

- Allow your chin to fall towards your chest. Now that your back is arched upward, gently push the range until you feel a nice stretch, but not so much you feel pain. Hold this for 5 to 10 seconds at the peak of your movement while breathing normally.
- Before transitioning to the next position, take a deep inhale.
- Exhale and allow your spine to extend at the same time, gently pushing your stomach towards the ground. Lift your head and tailbone, arching your back until you feel the stretch. Hold for 5 to 10 seconds at the peak of your movement while breathing normally.

As you gain flexibility and control over your core muscles, work to increase your comfortable range by pushing your back further to the ceiling and your stomach close to the ground on each inhale and exhale.

Building and maintaining a healthy, supported range in your spine is not only brilliant to improve and strengthen your posture, but it also plays an important part in protecting your intervertebral discs (among other things!), meaning you will be far less likely to suffer from back pain or incur injury.

This is such an incredibly important part of living an active and independent life that is often overlooked. As with all of the positions, movements, and poses in this book, it doesn't matter where you start. What matters is how you progress over the coming weeks.

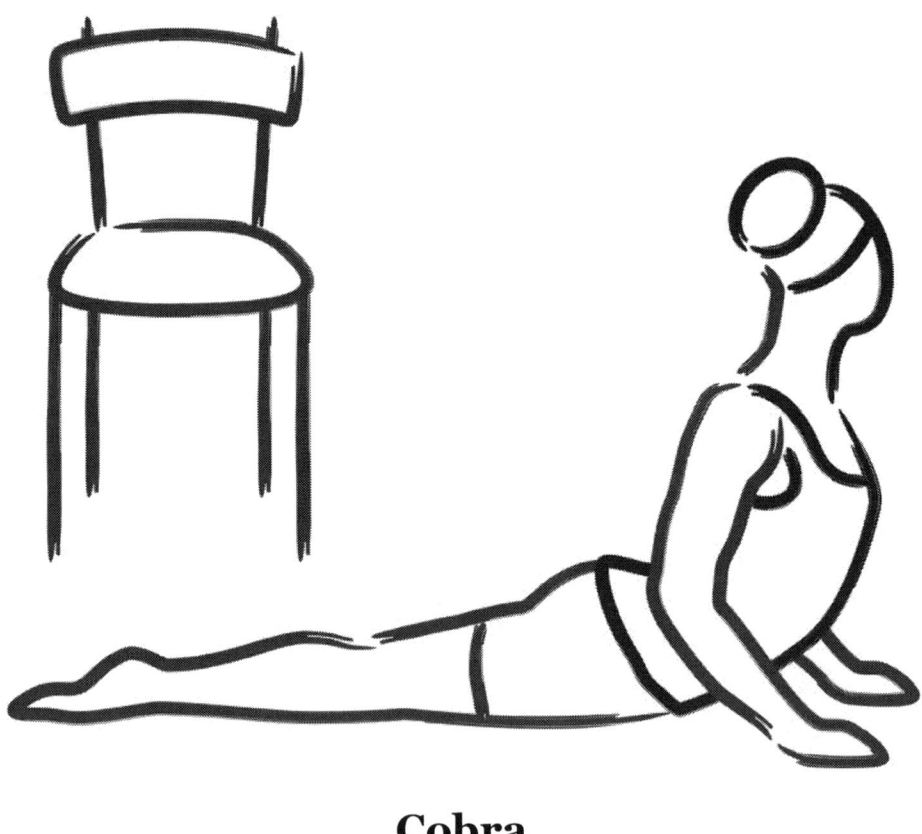

Cobra

Similar to the cat-cow, the cobra pose helps improve and maintain your spine's range, stability, and health. Its other benefits include that it helps to improve circulation, expand the lunges, and regulate the adrenal and thyroid glands (which are responsible for delivering essential hormones throughout your body).

How to get into a Cobra Pose:

- Lie face down on your mat. Keep your feet shoulder-width apart, and your toes pointed.
- Place your hands under your shoulders, with your elbows tucked into your body. Take a deep breath in.
- Slowly breathe out while straightening your arms and lifting your chest off of the ground. Let your hips hang downward, aiming to

keep as much of your thighs as you can in contact with the mat, to extend your spine.
- Once you reach the peak of your movement (pain-free range), draw your shoulders back and breathe normally.
- Hold the pose for up to 30 seconds before returning to your start position.
- Complete 1 to 5 repetitions.

Note:

When lifting yourself into position, stop straightening your arms when you feel your pelvis start to leave the mat. If you find that you are unable to extend your arms to begin with, start off on your elbows, focus on feeling a stretch through your abs and a comfortable extension in your spine.

This pose may look simple, but it requires a lot of arm strength, core stability, and spinal flexibility. There's no rush to reach maximum range. As good as these movements are for your spinal health, forcing yourself into a range that you're not quite ready for can have the opposite effect. The fastest way to progress is to move at a pace that works for you.

I like to use the following analogy: All exercise should be compared to building a house. When you take the time to build a solid foundation, the house will be strong. Skip building a solid foundation, and the house will collapse. With this in mind, take your time and build a foundation that will last a lifetime.

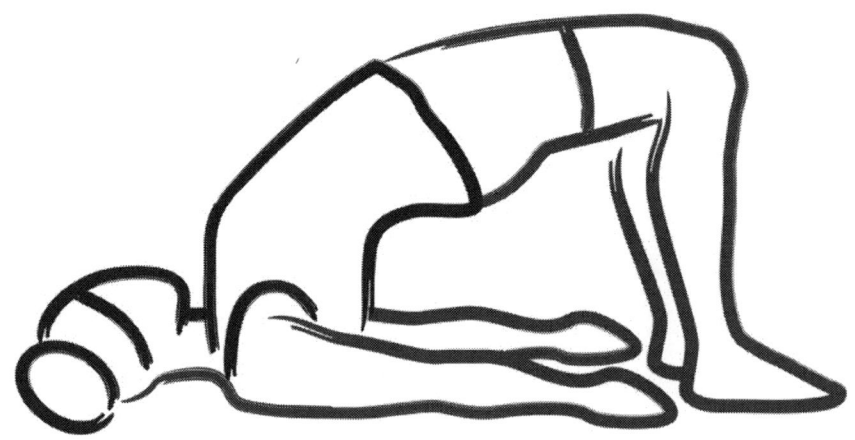

Glute Bridge

This simple but brilliant exercise increases strength and stability in your hips, lower back, thighs, and core. If you struggle with lower back or knee pain, this exercise will teach your body to take the pressure and strain away from those areas by putting more load into your glutes and core muscles.

Teaching your body how to properly engage and load your glutes and core together massively improves your stability in almost all movements in your daily life. Whether your movements involve squatting, walking, running, or balancing, glute strength and stability play a huge part.

How to get into a glute bridge:

- Lie down on your back. Bend your knees and root your feet flat on the ground, hip distance apart.
- Place your arms at your sides with your palms facing down.
- Now inhale.
- As you exhale, push up through the heels of your feet, lifting your hips until your knees, hips, and shoulders are in a straight line (for future reference, pushing your hips through like this is also known as 'finishing the hips'), all while keeping your shoulders and head on the ground.
- Brace your glutes (that means tense your buttocks!) and engage your core muscles by drawing your abs in.
- Hold for 10 seconds while breathing normally before lowering your hips back down to the ground.
- Repeat under control for 10 to 15 repetitions.

As you progress through the set, focus on your glutes to help strengthen your mind/muscle connection. As your glutes start to fatigue, you will feel them burn. This is normal and just shows that your target muscles (in this case, your glutes) are working correctly.

Notes:

To increase the difficulty, when you lower your hips to the ground, only allow about 20% of your weight down onto the floor between repetitions. This will increase the time that your muscles are under tension by removing that short rest period between reps.

FREE BONUS: CHAIR YOGA POSES PRINTABLE CHART

I have put together each of the pictured chair yoga poses from this chapter into an easy-to-follow video guide and a full color chart that you can print out. To get access, head over to bit.ly/chair-yoga-free in your internet browser, and I'll send it to you right away!

You can also scan the QR Code below with your cell phone camera and tap on the link that pops up if you find that easier.

I hope that this makes your workouts a little easier.

4

MORNING CHAIR YOGA ROUTINE

"Yoga is the cessation of the movements of the mind. Then there is abiding in the Seer's own form."

- PATANJALI

As you know, chair yoga can be used for more than just a workout. It can also be used to help release tension from the body, improve circulation, and help you start your day off on the right foot. Reserving ten to fifteen minutes in the morning for a chair yoga routine will help you get the most out of your day.

The Benefits of Stretching and Practicing Yoga in the Morning

A study in the 'Journal of Bodywork and Movement Therapies' found that practicing yoga helped improve your mood, improve energy levels, and reduce stress and anxiety. In a second study, yoga was found to improve your cognitive performance and make you more productive throughout the day.

With so many amazing benefits, it's no wonder that starting your day with a chair yoga routine comes so highly recommended. The main benefits of stretching and practicing yoga in the morning include:

- **Relieve back pain and tension**: Sleeping in the same position all night can cause tension in the back and shoulders. Stretching first thing in the morning using the right combination of chair yoga poses can help to relieve the tension and engage the body to start your day feeling good.
- **Improved circulation**: Chair yoga helps improve your circulation and is a low-impact way to warm up your joints and muscles first thing in the morning.
- **Switch on your balance**: By engaging your core muscles and firing up your hip stabilizers, you greatly improve your body's ability to automatically correct itself as a reflex. Switching on these important muscles first thing in the morning will help to prevent rolled ankles, unsteadiness, falls, and ultimately injury.
- **Improve your mood**: Even if you are not a morning person, you will find that practicing chair yoga can improve your mood and sense of well-being. Use it to energize you and fight off the crankiness you may feel when it's time to rise and shine.
- **Fight off stress and anxiety**: Aside from all forms of exercise being proven to release those feel-good endorphins, a few minutes of mindful breathing at the start and end of your chair yoga program will help to melt away any feelings of stress and anxiety.

- **Boost your metabolism**: Any form of exercise, especially first thing in the morning, has been proven to get your metabolism running hot. This is a great way to help your body burn through some extra calories.

Start Your Day Off Right

The aim of practicing chair yoga poses in the morning is to fully invigorate your body, switching on your core muscles and stabilizers, and to invigorate and energize you for the day, compared to the night chair yoga routine that is designed to help to calm the muscles and mind.

Note:

We have spent a fair amount of time in the previous chapters talking in depth about correct form, correct positions, how to engage your core muscles, upward and downward drivers, how to hinge and finish your hips, and so forth.

All of these teaching points are super important, and I would like you to keep them in mind as you progress through the rest of this book. In an attempt to stop myself from sounding too repetitive, I am going to assume that you've got a firm grasp and just use the key teaching points rather than continuing to talk at length.

With all that said, are you ready to get started in your morning chair yoga routine?

Here are the poses you can use to start your day off right:

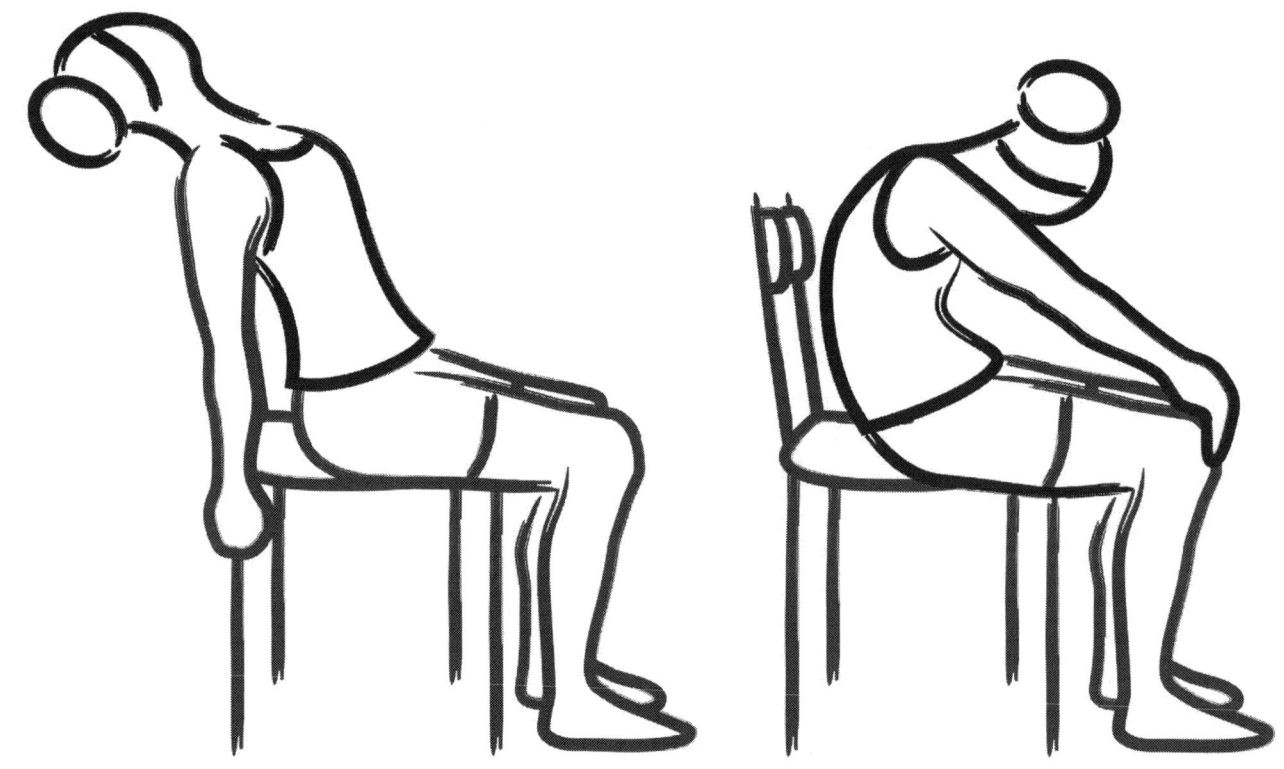

Seated Cat-Cow Stretch

Offering the same benefits as the cat-cow on all-fours, the seated cat-cow helps to improve dynamic range and mobility to the spine in the same way.

Follow these teaching points for a seated cat-cow:

- Sit upright, slightly forward on your chair, and with your feet planted hip distance apart. Now, take a deep breath in.
- Place your hands on either side of the seat behind you for support, lean back, and push your chest upward while breathing out. Draw

your shoulders back and downward as you feel your chest expanding.
- Hold this position for 5 to 10 seconds while breathing normally. This will allow your spine to extend to your current maximum range while stretching your chest.
- Slowly return to your start position.
- While sitting in an upright position, place your hands on your knees for support and take a deep breath in.
- Arch your back by pushing it towards the chair's backrest, tuck your hips, under and hand your head down. Breathing out as you move.
- Hold this position for 5 to 10 seconds while breathing normally. This will allow your spine to get into a controlled full flexion while stretching your mid-back and neck.
- Slowly return to your start position before repeating both movements for a further 5 to 8 repetitions.

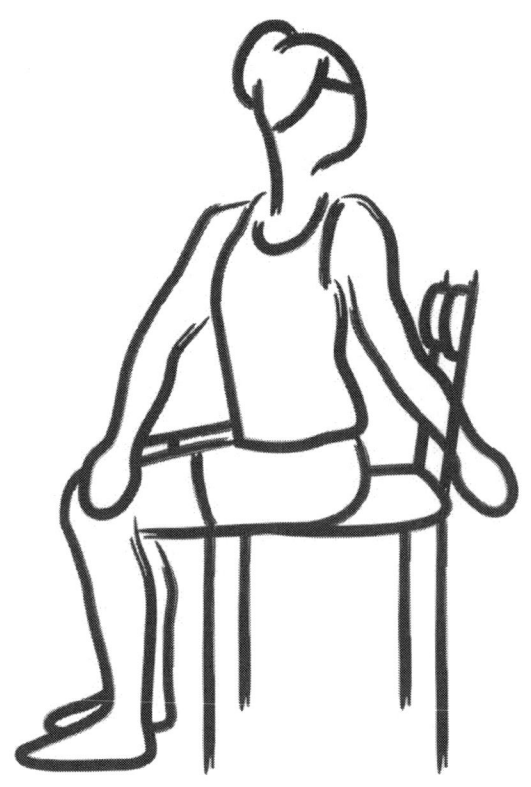

Seated Spinal Twist

The most obvious benefit of a seated spinal twist is to improve your rotational mobility. There is more to this simple position than you might think. As well as loosening your upper and lower back, it helps to stretch your chest, shoulders, and neck, which can be a big help in alleviating back and neck pain. It also improves circulation, tones your abs, and cleanses your organs.

Here's how:

- Start by sitting upright on your chair, with your feet planted on the ground shoulder distance apart and slightly away from your chair's backrest.
- We'll start by rotating to the left.
- Place your right hand across your lap and onto the outside of your left knee while allowing your left arm to hang by your side.
- Take a deep breath in.
- As you breathe out, rotate your body to the left, using your right arm against your left knee as leverage. If you would like to increase the leverage, you can use your left hand to grip the chair leg or backrest too.
- As you rotate, turn your head to the left and gently lift your chest.
- Hold the position for 10 to 20 seconds while breathing normally before returning to your start position and repeating on the opposite side.
- Repeat the seated spinal twists for 3-6 repetitions on each side.

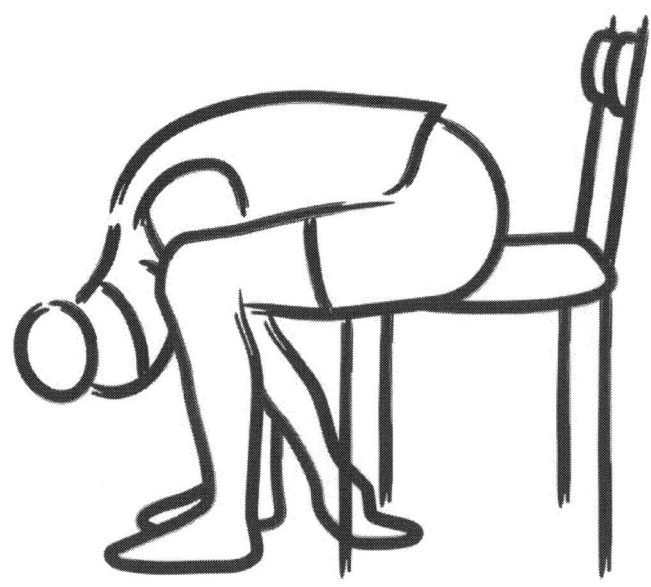

Full Range Seated Forward Folds

Alongside stretching your entire posterior chain, the seated forward fold is considered to be a stress-relieving, therapeutic posture, which is also good for reducing anxiety, centering the mind, and releasing fatigue.

Follow these teaching points and take your time to get the full benefit:

- Start by sitting in an upright position away from your chair's backrest, with your feet planted on the floor a little wider than shoulder width apart.
- Take a deep breath in.

- As you breathe out, hinge at your hips and allow your body to fold forward in a smooth and controlled action, aiming to hang your chest between your knees in a relaxed and pain-free position.
- Hang your arms downward, aiming to touch your fingertips on the floor. If you can already touch the floor, that's amazing! Try increasing the stretch by aiming your hands for a point on the floor behind you.
- Hold the stretch for 10-20 seconds while breathing normally.
- When you are ready to reset, take a deep breath in before you move.
- Now, smoothly unwind your body, slowly sitting up and lengthening your spine until you reach your start position. Remember to breathe out and activate your core as you move.
- Repeat for 3 to 5 repetitions.

Note:

Now that we're aiming for a deeper range of movement, you may experience a bit of a head rush as you practice this movement. If that does happen, return to your starting position and take controlled breaths until the feeling subsides. Reduce the range the next time you practice it.

There is a reduced range version of this pose described in Chapter 2 if you need to refresh your memory.

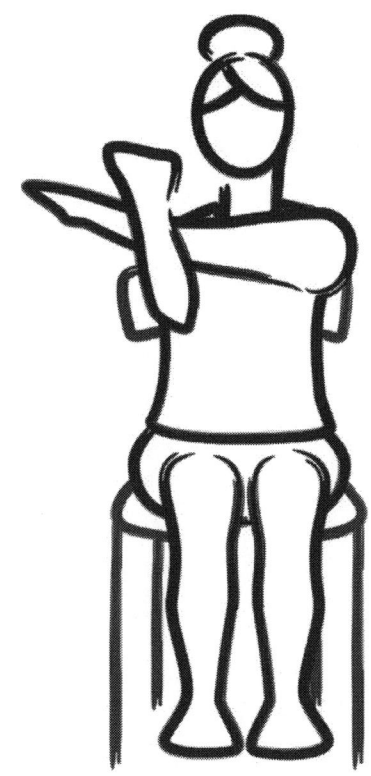

Seated Shoulder Stretch

Your shoulders take a lot of strain in your day-to-day life. They are constantly being loaded when you are carrying, lifting, and reaching, which can leave them tight and tired. By using a simple seated shoulder stretch, a lot of this tightness can be reduced quite easily.

Start out with just 15 seconds of resistance on one arm, then relax, and then repeat on the other arm.

To perform this stretch:

- Start by sitting upright on your chair.
- Take your left arm at shoulder height across your chest, aiming to keep it outstretched and soft at your elbow.

- Place your right hand behind your left upper arm, and gently apply a pulling pressure to it in a hugging action, drawing your outstretched target arm towards your chest.
- As you apply pressure, the shoulder of your target arm will begin to feel the stretch.
- Hold for up 30 seconds before repeating on your right.
- Repeat for 2 to 4 repetitions on each side.

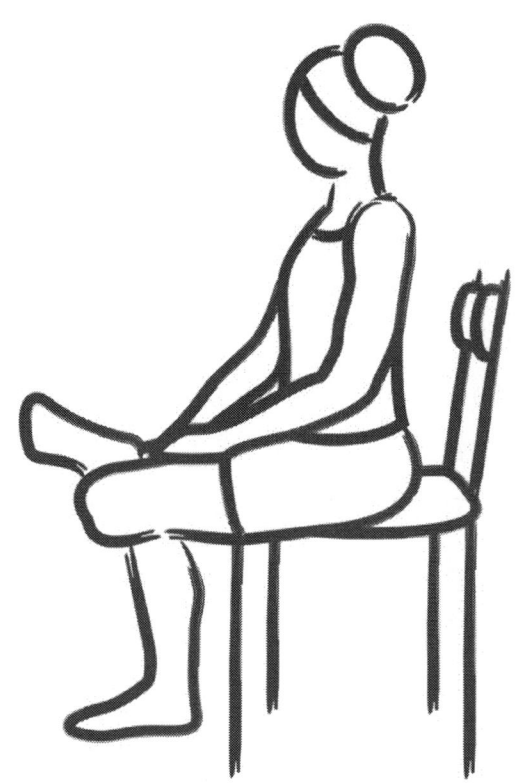

Seated Ankle-to-Knee Stretch

The ankle-to-knee stretch is a good way to give you a controlled but deep hip release helping you to build that all-important mobility.

I know that we have already looked at this stretch, but here's a reminder of the key teaching points:

- Sit upright on your chair and plant your feet flat on the ground.
- Rest your left ankle across your right knee and flare your left knee outward.
- Take a breath in. As you breathe out, allow your left knee to lower. To increase the stretch, gently push your left knee downward with your left hand.
- Hold this pose for 30 to 45 seconds before releasing the stretch and repeating it on the other side.

Note:

If you find that you don't have the flexibility to cross your ankle over your knee, that's no problem. Just cross the ankle of the leg that you are targeting the stretch, over your opposite ankle. Allow your knee to fall outward in the same way described in the teaching points, and gently use your hand to press your knee down and increase the stretch's intensity.

Improve at your own rate, and if that means that you start out with a reduced range version of any of these stretches or positions, that's totally fine. Don't worry about what level you start out at; focus on what level you want to get to instead. Also, think of it as a good measure of progress. Stay consistent with your chair yoga routines, and in just a few short weeks, you will see vast improvement. Think how good it will feel when you manage to complete a full set at full range of a movement that you found to be near impossible to begin with!

Focus on what you want, and keep up the good work.

FREE BONUS: CHAIR YOGA POSES PICTURE CHART

I have put together each of the pictured chair yoga poses from this chapter into an easy-to-follow video guide and a full color chart to that you can print out. To access these, head over to bit.ly/chair-yoga-free in your internet browser, and I'll send it to you right away!

You can also scan the QR Code below with your cell phone camera and tap on the link that pops up if you find that easier.

I hope that this makes your workouts a little easier.

5

EVENING CHAIR YOGA ROUTINE

"Energy and persistence conquer all things."

- BENJAMIN FRANKLIN

The versatility of chair yoga is really quite amazing. As we have already discussed, it can boost your metabolism and digestion, helping to manage body weight, it improves your mobility, strength, and balance, helping improve your muscle mass and joint health, and it can even be used to start your day on the right foot by getting you up and going in the morning.

In this chapter, we are going to look at how you can use chair yoga in the evening to help you unwind from the day. We will learn how to calm the mind and relax, which helps your body effectively recover and plays a very important part in maintaining both physical and mental health.

A good evening chair yoga routine can be used to chase off anxiety and help you let go of all the stresses from your day, giving you the best chance to slip into a restful and revitalizing sleep.

The Benefits of Practicing Yoga Before Bed

Chair yoga before bed provides many benefits for the mind and body. Here are some of the key benefits in a little more detail:

- **Fall asleep quicker**: Does it take you hours to fall asleep at night, no matter how exhausted you feel? The right chair yoga routine before bed will loosen the muscles and clear the mind, and it has been proven to make it easier for you to fall asleep. For those suffering from insomnia and other sleep problems, chair yoga may be the solution you've been looking for.
- **Better quality sleep**: Going to sleep quickly is only one piece of the puzzle. The quality of your sleep also matters. You could spend hours in bed and still feel exhausted when you wake. Why is this? One of the biggest reasons is that if you are unable to fall into enough deep REM sleep or if your body is stiff or sore, meaning that when you move while asleep, it disturbs your sleep cycle enough to pull you out of REM without waking you up, you are highly likely to rise but not shine in the morning. Yoga can help calm the mind, so you can find a deep sleep much faster and reduce joint and muscle stiffness to help you stay there.
- **Weight loss**: Chair yoga promotes weight loss both directly and indirectly. Your muscle mass directly governs the rate at which your metabolism burns calories both at rest and in motion. Therefore, the more quality muscle you have, the faster your metabolism is. Notice how many exercises in this book get your muscles working hard! Indirectly, chair yoga can be used to calm down and relax you at the end of the day; as mentioned above, it

helps you sleep better. This helps reduce stress, which in turn lowers the levels of cortisol in your bloodstream. While cortisol is a natural and vital hormone produced in the body as a response to stress, allowing its levels to build up over time can negatively impact you.

Cortisol is responsible for insulin release, inflammatory response, immune function, glucose metabolism, and blood pressure regulation, so all important stuff! The problem is that when it is released in high amounts for prolonged periods of time, all of these natural processes can get knocked off-track, which is not good for your health. Yoga helps to reduce cortisol levels, allowing your body to return to and maintain its natural balance.

- **Promotes relaxation**: Chair yoga is great for putting your body into a calm state of relaxation. During the day, you have many stressors that put you into a fight or flight response, adding tension to the body. One of the aims of an evening chair yoga routine is to help lower blood pressure and relax the whole body.

Simple Evening Chair Yoga Poses

As you can see from the benefits above, the aim of practicing chair yoga in the evening is to fully unwind your body, release stress and tension, and help you enter a state of relaxation, making it easier to slip into a deep and restful sleep.

To achieve this state, I have found that the following selection of poses works incredibly well:

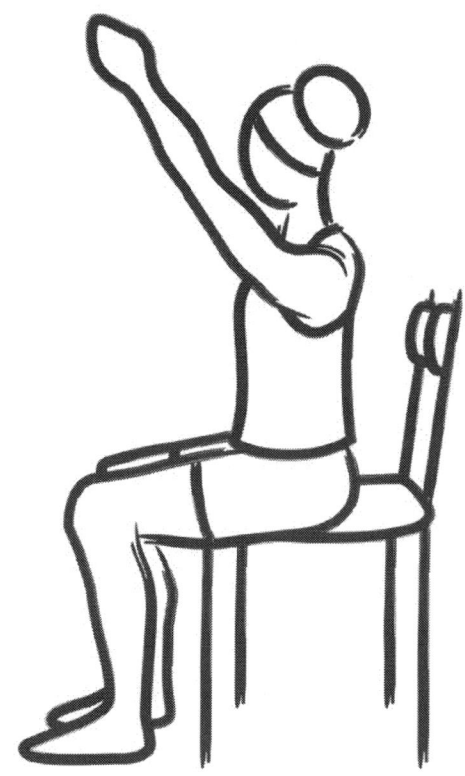

Seated Urdhva Hastasana

The main goal of the Urdhva Hastasana pose is to loosen up the muscles around your shoulder blades and relieve tension in the upper back and neck. Your aim is to reach your arms above your head and stretch towards the ceiling. If you have limited mobility in your shoulders and arms, the movement can be easily adapted to suit your current flexibility level.

- Start by sitting upright in your chair with your feet hip distance apart. Now, take a breath in.
- With your arms stretched out ahead of you, slowly reach forwards and then overhead until you are at the peak of your range while breathing out.

- Once at the peak of your range, stretch upward until you can feel your mid-back around your shoulder blades stretching.
- Hold this stretch for 20 seconds while breathing normally.
- Breath in. Now, release the stretch and then slowly lower your arms down in front of you and then down to your sides while breathing out.
- Take a moment before repeating for 4 to 8 repetitions.

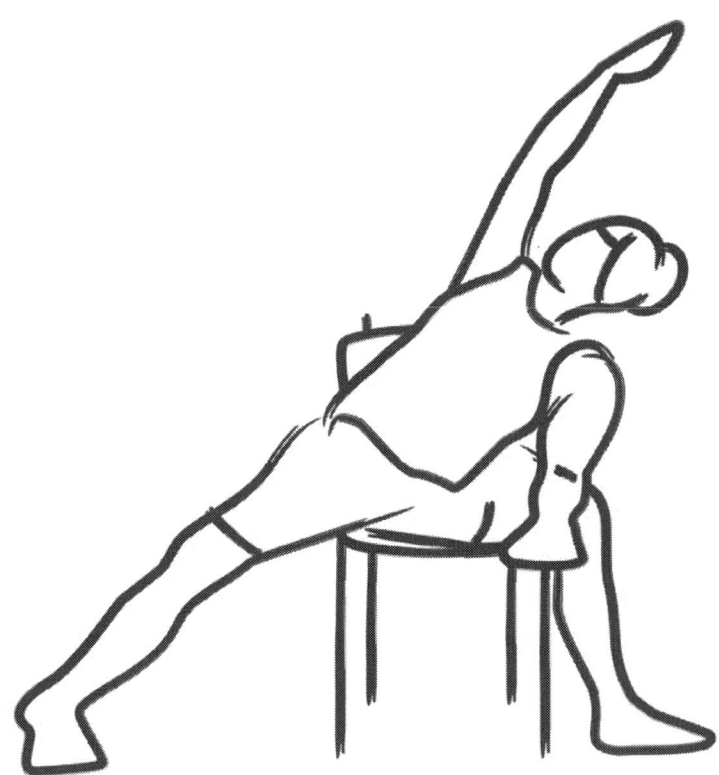

Chair Extended Side Angle

As we have discussed this pose in detail earlier, let's get straight to the teaching points:

- Start by sitting in an upright position in your chair.

- Keeping your left knee flexed at 90 degrees, rotate your hips to the left, and face your left foot out to the side.
- Hinge your hips, fold your body forward towards your left knee, and lean your left arm on top of your left thigh for support.
- Extend your right leg out to the opposite side until straight (remain soft at the knee). Adjust your right foot so it's flat on the floor and faces forward. Take a breath in.
- Rotate your body to the right and extend your right arm overhead to expand your chest. As you reach overhead, breathe out.
- Hold for 10 to 20 seconds and breathe normally.
- Return to your start position and then repeat on the opposite side.
- Complete 3-6 repetitions on each side.

This pose works well to relieve any built-up tension being held in your back, neck, and shoulders. If you would like to increase the stretch further, reach the arm that you would normally rest on your thigh and reach it down towards the floor until you're able to touch your fingertips down.

When you feel ready to progress your mobility to the next level, consider making your first two repetitions of your set as described in the teaching points above before adding the extra range. This will help to get your body used to the movement and locks your form in before you push yourself further.

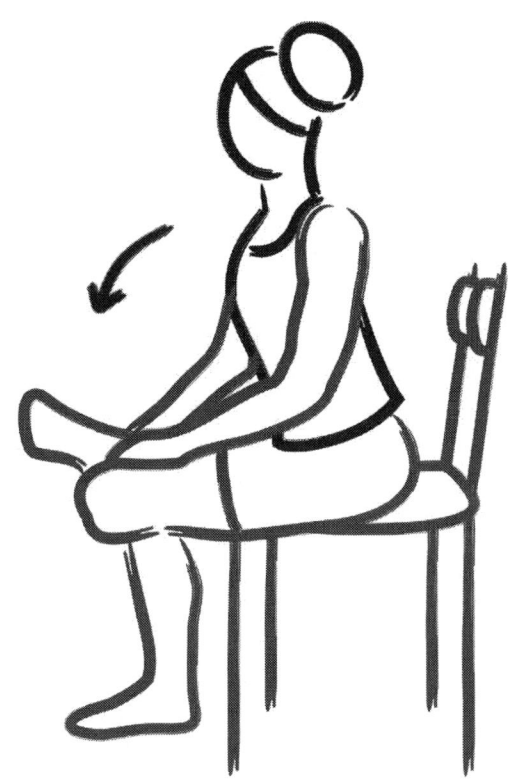

Chair Pigeon

Here are the key teaching points to help you get the most out of the chair pigeon pose. For a more in-depth look, refer to Chapter 2:

- Sit upright on your chair with your feet hip distance apart.
- Cross your left leg over your right, resting your left ankle on your right thigh. Take a breath in.
- As you breathe out, hinge at your hips and tip your body forward to increase the stretch in your hip and glute.

Side Note: So many people suffer from lower back or knee discomfort due to reduced range in their hips. The reason is that when the hip loses range, strength, and stability (or, in some cases, all three!), your body will make up for what it's lost by adding the extra load to the next thing in your body's movement chain. So, in the case of your hips, it will either travel upward to your lower back or downward to your knees! The hip is classed as one of the 'three rocks' of the body, the others being the foot/ankle and the thoracic spine (upper spine, not including the neck).

The aim of this pose is to feel the stretch along the hip and thigh muscles. As you gain flexibility, you can increase range and the stretch's intensity by gently pushing the crossed-over leg a little. As you gain muscular endurance, it will become easier to hold the stretch.

More Side Notes: Rather than sounding like a science manual and droning on, I have tried to keep explanations short and sweet so that you can get everything you need from your chair yoga programs as efficiently as possible. If you're interested in finding out more about the three rocks of the body and their functions, head to bit.ly/chair-yoga-free in your internet browser and, I will send you an email in the coming week explaining it in more detail.

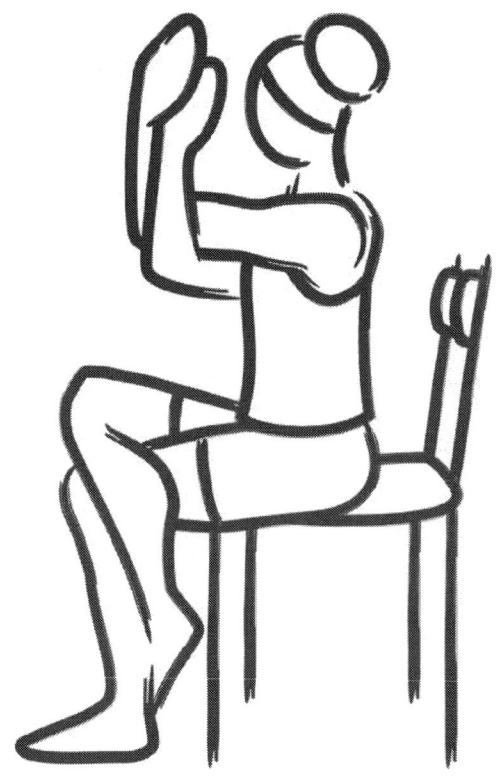

Chair Eagle

Earlier in the book, we discussed this tricky intertwining pose in detail. All chair yoga poses require practice in order for you to really get the most out of them, especially when they require a lot of range of motion and coordination. Please focus on the following teaching points to help you get into the chair eagle pose. If you need to refresh your memory on the more detailed points, please refer to Chapter 2:

- Sit upright on your chair with your feet hip distance apart.
- Cross your right leg over your left and hook your right foot back around your left ankle in a winding motion. If you don't quite have

EVENING CHAIR YOGA ROUTINE

the range for this yet, take your right leg to a point where you feel a comfortable stretch for now with the view to increasing range as your flexibility improves.

- Now, raise your arms in front of you and cross your left arm over your right.
- Fold at the elbows so that both your arms point upward. Your goal is to wind your arms around themselves until your palms touch together. Just like with your legs, if you don't quite have the range for this yet, take it the point that you feel a comfortable stretch, with a view to increasing your range a little more each day.
- Now active your core muscles, lift your chest, and breathe normally.
- Hold the pose for 30 to 60 seconds.
- Return to your start position before repeating the pose on the opposite side.

Note:

Take your time, concentrate on executing all your poses with good form, and once you're holding the pose, focus on what you're trying to target. This will ensure that you will always get the most out of your chair yoga programs.

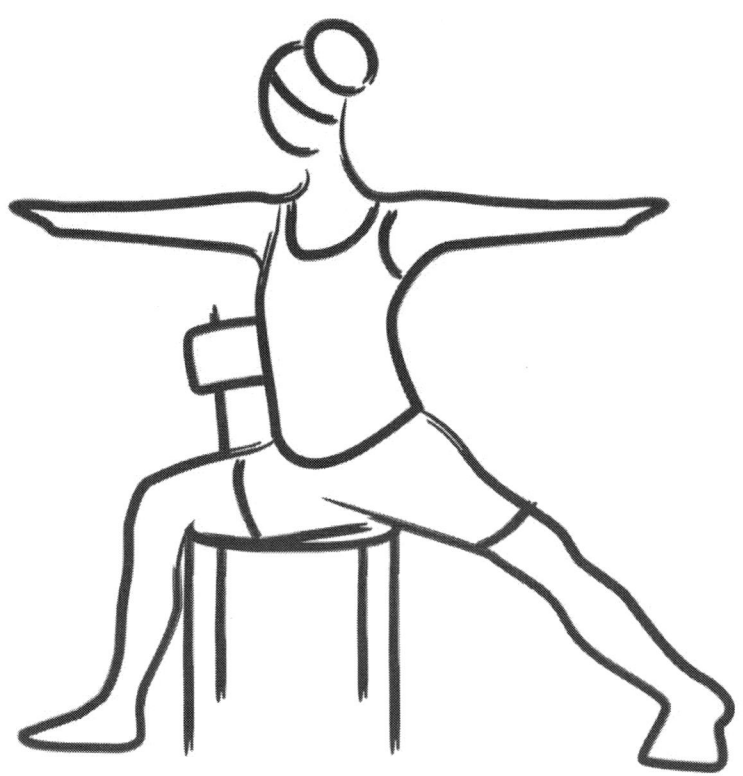

Chair Warrior II

I am a big fan of all the chair warrior poses. As one of my lovely clients once told me, "They just look so yoga". That line has always stuck with me, and I couldn't have put it better myself!

Here are the key teaching points for the chair warrior II pose:

- Start sitting upright on your chair, slightly over to the left-hand side of the seat.
- Turn to your right and get into a high lunge position, making sure that your right leg is supported by the chair and your left is outstretched behind.

- Turn the foot on your outstretched leg to face forward, making sure that you keep it flat on the ground. Only turn it as far as you can while remaining stable and comfortable. Take a breath in.
- Raise both arms, one in front and one behind, to shoulder height. Open your chest, lengthen your neck, and breathe out as you move. Focus on drawing your shoulder blades back and down.
- Hold the pose for 30 seconds while breathing normally.
- Now release the pose and transition either to the opposite side or onto the next pose.

Note:

You can practice the chair warrior II pose on one side and then the other, or you can transition straight from your chair warrior II pose into the next pose on the program (the reverse chair warrior pose) and then switch to the other side.

Flowing from one pose straight into the next on your program can be a great way to build your skill level, your coordination, and your core stability. Despite these extra benefits, I want you to think of this as a 'nice if I do' rather than an 'I have to do' part of your program.

I'll leave that up to you.

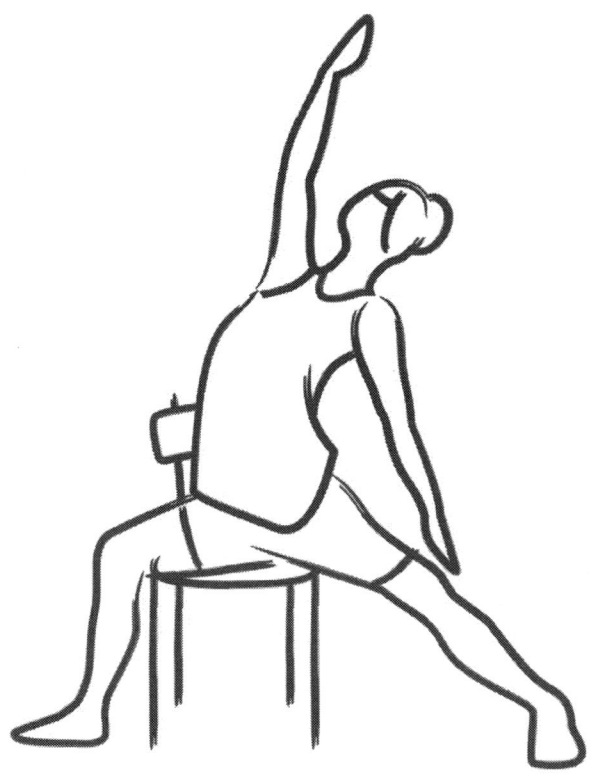

Reverse Chair Warrior

Whether you're flowing into this pose directly from the previous one on your program or practicing it as an individual movement, the reverse chair warrior is a fantastic way to help you finish your chair yoga program with a sense of relaxation but also empowerment.

To find the correct position, start out in the chair warrior II pose and then follow these key teaching points:

- While in a right-facing chair warrior II pose, take a deep breath in.
- Now breathe out and lower your left arm towards your outstretched left leg while raising your right arm toward to the ceiling. Focus on using both arms as downward drivers to help extend your spine as you move.

EVENING CHAIR YOGA ROUTINE

- Hold this position for 20 to 30 seconds while breathing normally.
- Release the pose and practice on the opposite side.

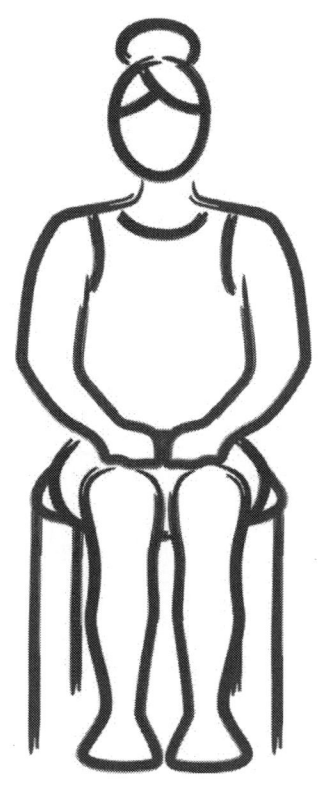

Seated Savasana

Once you complete your evening chair yoga routine, I would like you to sit in an upright posture against your chair's backrest, plant your feet on the ground, hips distance or narrower apart, place your hands in your lap, close your eyes, breathe normally, and take a moment.

This is your chance at the end of your chair yoga session to let the stretches and poses that you have worked through work their magic as your body embraces any newfound range of movement.

If you're a visual person, I would like you to picture a single candle in front of you. Imagine that each time you breathe in, your breath draws the candle flame towards you, and when you breathe out, the flame gently moves away.

You've learned a lot and have come a long way since you first picked up this book. Now that you have practiced and understand a wide array of chair yoga positions, poses, and key points, you are ready to progress onto your 21-day chair yoga program.

I'm proud of the progress you've made so far. Now, let's hold our focus and keep the good work going.

FREE BONUS: CHAIR YOGA POSES PRINTABLE CHART

I have put together each of the pictured chair yoga poses from this chapter into an easy-to-follow video guide and a full color chart to that you can print out.

For access to these, head over to bit.ly/chair-yoga-free in your internet browser, and I'll send it to you right away!

You can also scan the QR Code below with your cell phone camera and tap on the link that pops up if you find that easier.

I hope that this makes your workouts a little easier.

6

BEGINNER CHAIR YOGA PROGRAM DAY 1 - 7

"A little progress each day adds up to big results."

- SATYA NANI

You have come a long way since you first picked up this book. Now that you understand the basic how and whys of chair yoga, it is time for you to put it into practice and begin your first 21-day routine.

Why 21 days, you may ask? The simple answer is that 21 days is a short enough amount of time to stay focused on your goal while being long enough to see a real change in your strength, mobility, and balance. Another great reason is that it takes a minimum of 18 days to form a new habit, so after 21 days of following a properly phased program, it will feel far easier to make chair yoga a part of your healthy daily life.

The following three chapters will walk you through 3 x 7-day programs. We shall start your 21-day program with a 7-day beginner level program, progressing on to a 7-day intermediate level program, and finishing on a 7-day advanced level.

I have structured the following 21 days in this way so you will feel yourself progressing measurably each week and so that you can achieve the most results out of the shortest amount of time by making it progressively tougher as you improve to keep increasing your muscle flexibility and joint mobility, your muscle strength and joint stability, your balance and core strength.

This doesn't mean that if you don't feel ready to tackle the advanced program on week three of your first 21 days, that's no problem at all. You can still achieve fantastic results by simply switching out the program you don't feel ready for yet, and repeat the previous week's program for 7 more days.

For example:

Your first run-through of your 21-day program may look something like this.

- Day 1 – 7: Beginner
- Day 8 – 14: Beginner
- Day 15 – 21: Intermediate

And your second run through like this:

- Day 1 – 7: Intermediate
- Day 8 – 14: Intermediate
- Day 15 – 21: Advanced

As long as you practice consistently and focus on progressing a little more each day, you'll do great. Don't think of your chair yoga journey as a race to progress. The most important things are that you maintain good form, feel it where you are supposed to, and push yourself just enough so that your body has no choice but to adapt to the overload you place upon it.

The following program is an effective starting place for the next 21 days and suitable for beginners; along with some of the modifications we discussed in previous chapters, you can increase the difficulty level day by day by adding depth, range, extra repetitions, and hold times as you feel your strength growing, your stability improving, and your flexibility increasing. Some of the poses are new to us, but the work we have already covered in the previous chapters has more than prepared you for them.

You should be proud of the progress you've made so far. Now, let's get to it and keep the good work going!

Days 1 to 7

Warm Up Your Body and Connect with Your Breath

Before we begin, take a moment to warm up your body and connect with your breath. You only need to spend two or three minutes on this, but it will ensure that you get the maximum benefit out of your session.

Start out by running through the dynamic stretches we practiced in Chapter 1 (you can print the dynamic stretch sheet out if it makes it easier for you to follow; just scan the QR code at the end of the previous chapter).

Once you have warmed your body up, it's time to take a seat, take control of your breathing, and focus on making it nice and steady.

If you're not sure, here are some tips on how you can connect with your breath:

- Sit upright in your chair and close your eyes while maintaining good posture.
- Take a deep breath in through your nose over a count of 3 before exhaling out of your mouth for a count of 4 or 5.
- Place your hands on your stomach, feeling it expand as you breathe in and deflate as you breathe out.

With each inhale, notice the coolness of your breath when it starts to hit your nostrils. As you exhale, feel the warmth of the breath leaving the body. This helps to focus your mind, control your heart rate, and prepare your body.

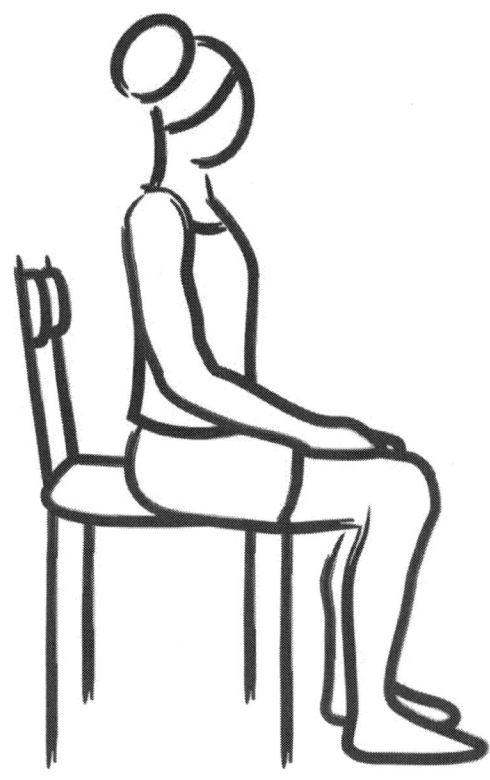

Mountain Pose

When you are ready, it is time to adjust your posture into a mountain pose. This helps open your chest, lengthen your spine, and activate your core and upper back muscles.

To transition into mountain pose:

- Sit up tall in your chair with your feet hip distance apart.
- Gently press your tailbone downward into the chair while elongating your neck and body. Imagine that there's a piece of string attached to the top of your head that is being gently drawn up.
- Place your hands on your lap and draw your shoulder blades back and down to open your chest. Try to imagine that you're gripping an invisible pencil between the bottom of your shoulder blades.

- Activate your core muscles by slightly drawing in your abs, and hold your position for 20 to 30 seconds while practicing your controlled breathing.

If you'd like to increase the stretch in your chest, you can tuck your hands behind your lower back.

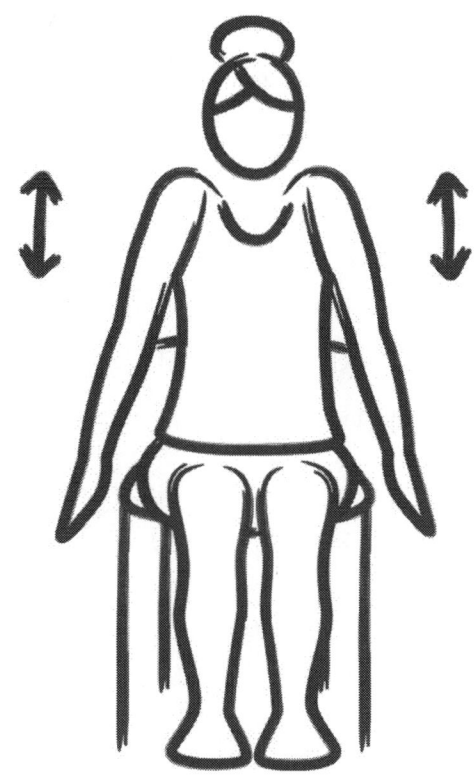

Shoulder Shrug and Release

Now that your body muscles and joints are warm and your breathing is steady, you can start with the main movements of your program, starting with a shoulder shrug and release.

The main benefits include, improved posture and neck stability, increased strength in your shoulders and upper trapezius (the top of your shoulder where the straps of a backpack would sit) and range, and improved upper body circulation.

Here are the key teaching points:

- Sit upright in a mountain pose (the previous position).
- Inhale slowly and shrug your shoulders up toward your ears while squeezing them back. Hold at the top until you finish inhaling.
- Exhale slowly and push your shoulders down while drawing them back. When you reach your full range, focus on elongating your neck. Hold position until you finish your exhale.
- Repeat for 10 to 15 repetitions.

When you reach the topmost point of your shrug, you will feel your upper spine extend, and as you reach your full range on the way down, you should feel your neck lengthen, all while working your back and shoulder muscles.

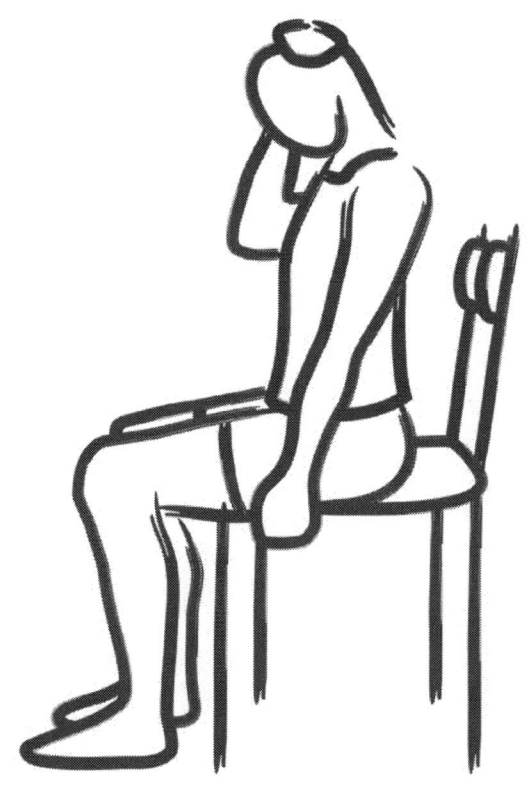

Ear-to-Shoulder Neck Stretch

Now that you have exercised your shoulders and neck, it's time to work on its lateral flexion (side bend). This stretch will help build up controlled range in your neck and thoracic spine, which helps keep your posture stable, reduces neck pain and stiffness, and can even reduce tension headaches! Like always, take your time and push yourself until you feel a comfortable, controlled stretch. The more often you practice, the quicker your range will improve, and the rewards will come.

To get the most out of your ear-to-shoulder neck stretch, follow these teaching points:

- Sit upright in your chair. Before you stretch, set your shoulders by first lifting them and then rolling them back and down. This will ensure they are in the correct position when you apply the stretch.
- Look straight ahead, centering your neck position, and hang both arms at your sides.
- Hook your right hand over the top of your head, allowing the middle finger of that hand to touch the top of your left ear while flaring your right elbow out to the side. Take a deep inhale.
- As you exhale, gently tip your head to the right, aiming your right ear toward your right shoulder. Move slowly and smoothly, allowing the weight of your right arm to carry you into the stretch.
- Hold the position for 5 deep breaths. Each time you breathe out, try to relax further, allowing the weight of your stretching arm to carry your neck to your current range on its own before gently releasing the stretch and returning your head to its centered position.
- Complete the stretch on the opposite side before repeating for 3 to 5 repetitions on each side.

By allowing the weight of your arm to stretch your neck and letting gravity do the work for you, you will only ever take it as far as your current range allows. Never pull or jerk while stretching, as this will force your body to resist and can have negative consequences. Be confident with your movements while applying them all with smooth control.

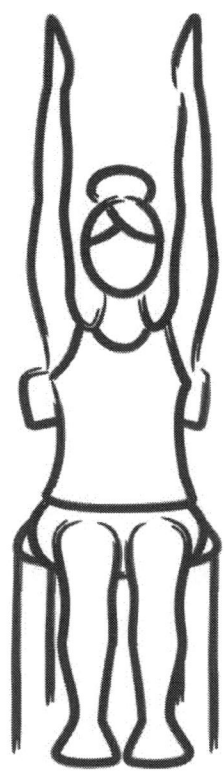

Front Arm Lifts

The next movement focuses on toning the arms while mobilizing the shoulders and thoracic spine. Before you begin, get yourself into the mountain pose and then follow the teaching points:

- Extend both arms out straight in front of you with your palms facing each other.
- Inhale and lift both arms overhead, stretching upward as you reach the peak of your movement. Focus on keeping your posture in a neutral position and your core engaged while you move.
- Exhale and lower both arms back out in front of you. This will keep your muscles engaged for the whole set. If you feel that you need a

moment's rest between repetitions, simply lay your hands in your lap for a moment before continuing your set.
- Complete 10 to 15 repetitions before taking a 30 to 45 seconds rest.
- Repeat for 2 more sets.

Ideally, you will be able to reach directly overhead while maintaining good posture. If you find that you are unable to reach full range to begin with, don't worry; just work to your current range with the view of increasing it a little more each day.

It's also worth mentioning; if you find that your range decreases as your muscles become fatigued, that's actually a good thing! It shows that you're pushing yourself to work hard. Finish all the sets with a slightly reduced range so you can maintain the form.

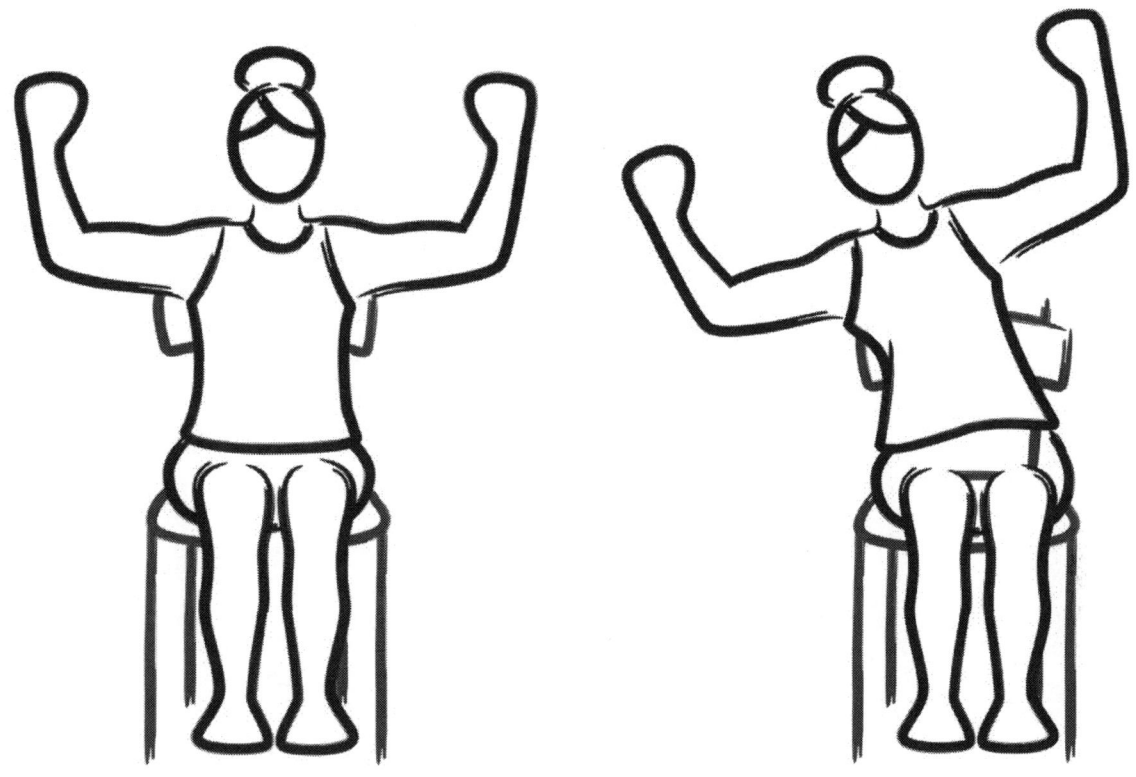

Side Bend with Arms in Cactus Position

This movement offers a variety of benefits. The cactus position helps lengthen and strengthen your rotator cuff muscles. The rotator cuff is primarily responsible for the stability of the ball and socket part of your shoulder joint. The cactus position helps build strength and stability by laterally rotating it (rotating your arm away from your center line) and then bracing it. This position also builds strength and range in your back by lengthening your thoracic spine at the same time.

I have put the cactus position together with a side bend so that you can also build lateral flexion through your entire spine rather than just your lumbar region (lower back). Building strength, range, and stability through your entire spine, massively improves the way that your whole body is supported as it moves in day-to-day life.

As you practice, try to envisage how each chair yoga pose and movement has a positive knock-on to what you do every day. Just one example of how having a strong and stable spine and shoulders can save you from injury: imagine you're standing on the bus, and suddenly, it breaks hard and jolts. If your back and shoulders are strong and stable, the jolt may take you by surprise but is unlikely to cause you an injury or fall.

I have broken the movement in two so that you can first get your arms in the correct position before moving on to practice the full movement; follow these teaching points in order:

- Start out in the mountain pose. Inhale and bring your arms up to shoulder height and out to your sides. Fold at your elbows, pointing your fingers straight up like goalposts, with your palms facing forward.
- Once your arms are in position, gently draw your shoulder blades back and down while lengthening your neck, and take a deep breath in.
- Exhale slowly. As you breathe out, smoothly bend your upper body to the right while focusing on keeping core muscles engaged. Even though you are controlling the movement, let gravity do its work to increase your stretch.
- You'll notice here that your arms and upper body are acting as a downward driver to your spine, so go slow!

- Hold the position for 5 controlled breaths before smoothly returning to your centered position. Take a moment before repeating the movement on the opposite side.
- Once you have completed on both sides. bring your arms together in front of you for a moment to relax your muscles before repeating for 5 another 2 to 4 repetitions.

During this whole set, keep your feet planted on the ground. If, for any reason, you feel unstable or as if the chair might tip, go back to your center position, plant your feet on the ground wider apart, and try again.

If you need to totally rest in between repetitions, that's no problem at all. Just place your hands in your lap and connect with your breath for up to 10 breaths before repeating.

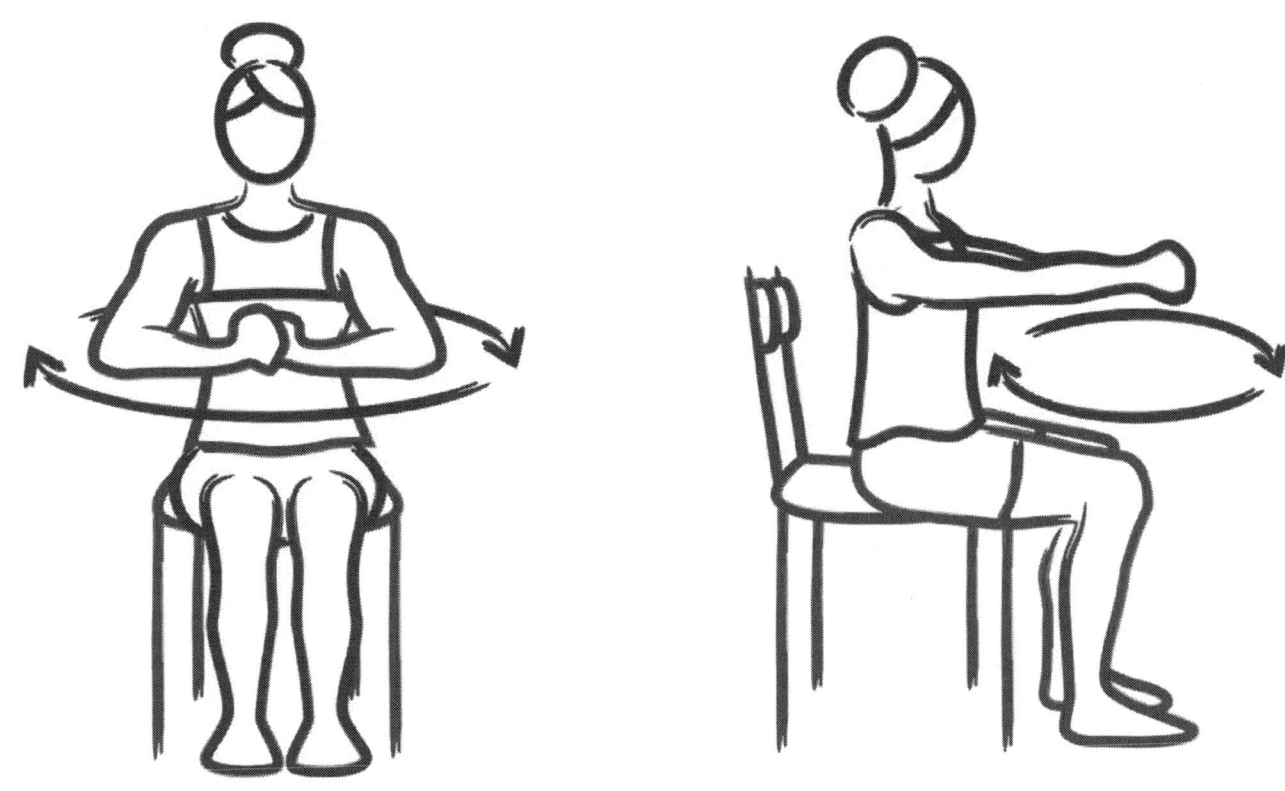

Stir the Pot

This movement combines your spine's mobility, core stability, and hip stabilizers, all while toning your arms.

The following teaching points run you through what to do:

- Start in a mountain pose with your feet narrow. If you want to decrease the difficulty, move your feet further apart to make you more stable.
- Make a fist with one hand and grasp it in the other like you're holding an imaginary ladle in both hands, with your arms out in front of you at chest height.

- In a horizontal stirring motion, circle your arm and allow your spine to move as you do. Focus on activating your core muscles by drawing your abs in and maintaining the same hand height throughout.
- Connect your breath with each stirring movement, breathe out as you stir outward, and breathe in as you stir inward.
- Complete 5 to 10 controlled repetitions in each direction for 4 sets.

As an added bonus, if you want to increase the difficulty further, try squeezing your hands together as you move. This will cause your chest muscles to activate isometrically.

This kind of movement is used a lot in martial arts such as tai chi and is believed to promote calming energy and mental clarity.

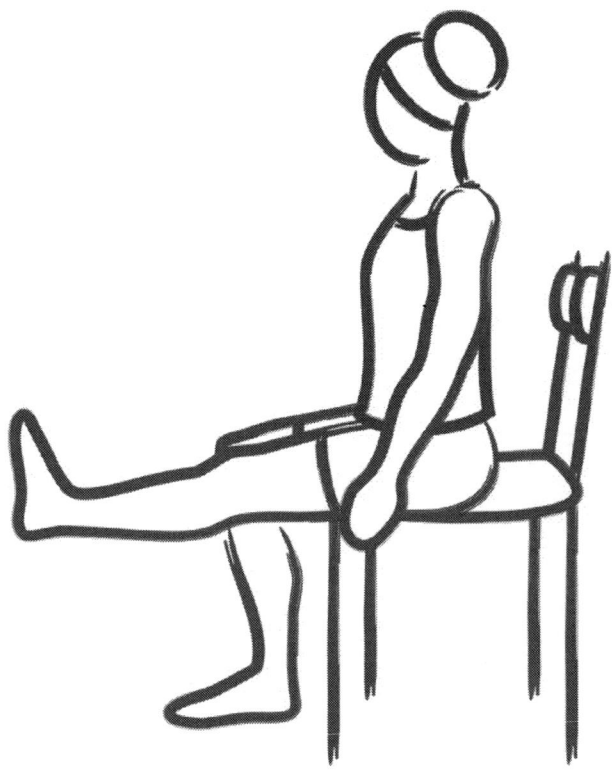

Leg Extension

Through this program, we have worked your body from the top down, putting a lot of focus on your shoulders, spine, and core. I would still like you to maintain a strong posture and a good level of core activation while we progress to work on your legs.

The seated leg extension puts focus on your quadricep muscles (the front of your thigh). The main purpose of this powerful muscle group is to extend your knee, but it is also responsible for stabilization as you stand, assisting with hip strength and stability, and absorbing impact force as your heel strikes the ground when you walk, all to keep you strong and to prevent injury.

Compared to many of the chair yoga poses and movements that we have already practiced together, this one is pretty simple, but to get the absolute most out of it, it's worth running through the teaching points:

- Start out in mountain pose with your feet hip distance apart and your core muscles fully engaged. Now, breathe in.
- We will start with your left leg. Extend your right leg until you feel your quadriceps (that's the muscle on the front of your thigh) squeezing and breathing out as you move.
- Hold for 3 to 5 breaths before slowly returning to your start position with both feet on the floor. Then, repeat for 10 repetitions on the same leg.
- Once you complete your 10 repetitions, switch to the opposite side.
- Repeat for 3 to 5 sets on each side, taking 10 to 30 seconds rest in between sets.

As you run through this exercise, you will notice that your quadricep is engaging when you extend your leg and will likely start to feel the burn as you complete your reps and sets. As your muscle becomes fatigued (and it will!), your range might start to decrease a little. If this happens, focus on maintaining your posture and core activation, even if that means reducing your range of movement a little. This will ensure that your target muscles do the work rather than placing unwanted strain elsewhere on your body.

The first few times you practice a leg extension, try placing your hand on your thigh to feel the muscular contraction as you move. This will help to reinforce your mind/muscle connection.

Note:

If you find that you are unable to fully extend your leg to begin with, that's fine. As long as you can feel your quadricep engaging during each repetition, you are doing well. As your legs become stronger, your muscular endurance improves, and your range increases over the coming week, you will be able to lift your leg to full range for every rep.

If completing full sets on each side feels too uncomfortable to begin with, try alternating legs after each rep. This is slightly easier on the legs, but it will still give you a lot of the benefits.

Optional:

If you feel brave enough and would like an extra challenge, after you have completed your leg extensions on both sides, try extending both legs at once to help activate the core (similar to a boat pose). Even an inch off the ground can help activate the core and lower body muscles.

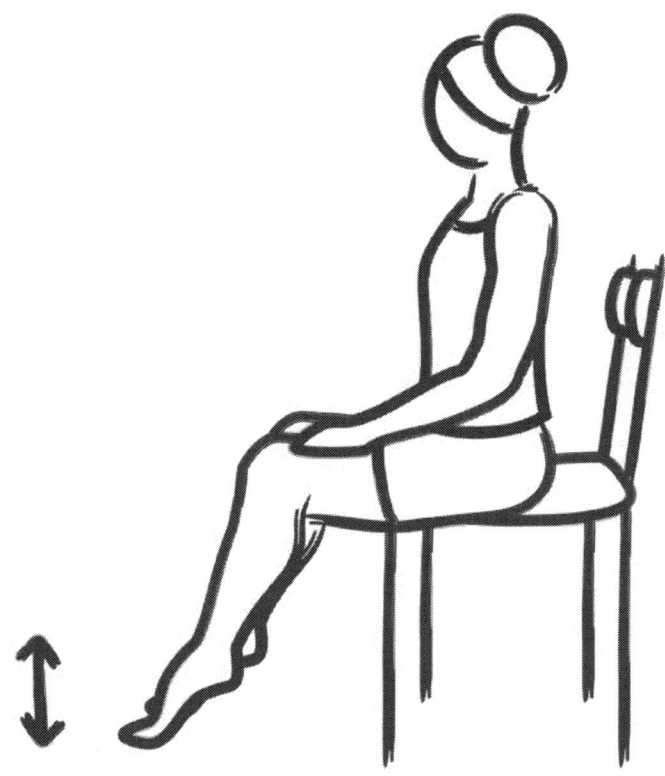

Calf Raises

To complete your beginner chair yoga program, I would like to bring focus to your calves and ankles. Your calves (the muscle group at the back of your lower leg) and your tibialis anterior (the opposing muscles to your calves that run down your shins) play a super important part in driving you forward as you walk and run, stabilizing you as you stand and move, and taking pressure away from your knees when you by absorbing impact, similar to a car's shock absorbers.

Calf raises are a simple exercise you can do from your chair, and they will work to build the range and balance mentioned above. Even though it's simple to get right, this movement makes a big difference to an active person's life. I have included the basic calf raise technique as well as some adaptations to build your strength through range even further. I suggest that you start by trying the base version first, and when you feel ready, move on from there.

Seated calf raise teaching points:

- Sit upright in your chair away from the backrest with your feet hip distance apart and both feet facing forward.
- Driving up through the balls of your feet, raise your heels off of the ground to your current maximum range. When you are at the peak of your range, you will feel your calves squeezing and a slight stretch running down your shins. Hold this squeezed position for 2 breaths before gently lowering your heels back to the floor.
- Make sure that you keep your core muscles activated as you move to help maintain a strong posture.
- Complete 10 to 15 controlled repetitions before taking a 30-second rest.
- Repeat for 3 sets.

When you feel ready to increase the difficulty, I would like you to start by adding some extra range to your movement.

- Complete 1 full repetition of a calf raise.
- Once your heels touch down, continue the movement by raising your toes off of the ground using your heels as a pivot point. When your toes are raised, you will feel the tibialis anterior (the muscle on your shin) contract and your calf stretch.

- Hold and squeeze this position for 2 breaths before lowering your toes back to the floor before repeating the whole calf raise to toe raise again for a full set of 10 to 15 repetitions.

Now that you have increased the range of movement in your ankles, let's increase the overload as an extra bonus:

- Place a weight onto your thighs and hold it in place with your hands. If you own some dumbbells, that's great; if not, you can use a backpack or bag with several bottles of water in it. I love using bottles of water in a bag as it's inexpensive and the weight can be adjusted.

Building strength through range in the calves and ankles is often overlooked, but they play such a vital role in maintaining an active life as we age.

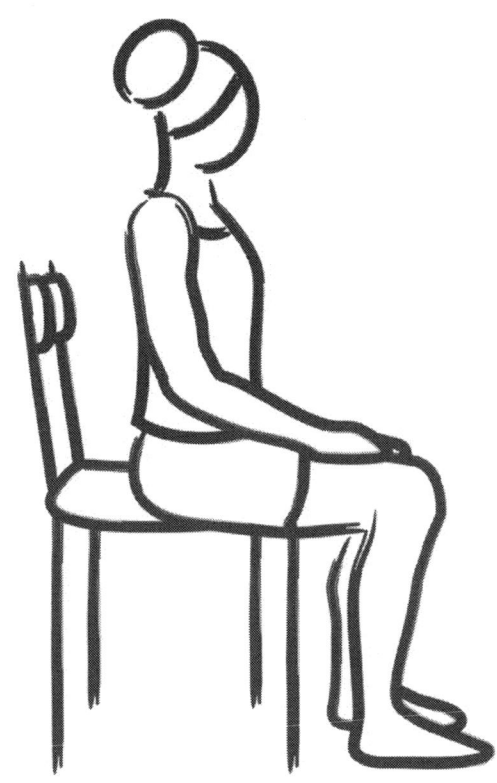

Seated Relaxation

After you have completed your chair yoga program, I recommend that you take 2 to 3 minutes to allow your body to unwind and recover before continuing your day. The practice of relaxation and mindfulness plays an important part in keeping your mind and body in balance.

So, before you wrap up your exercise session, follow these teaching points:

- Like at the beginning of the program, sit upright in a mountain pose. Close your eyes and connect with your breath.
- Focus on the effect your chair yoga poses and movements have had on your mind and body.
- Listen to your heart beating.

- Think about what parts of your session you feel you completed well and what parts you will focus on improving next time.
- Allow yourself to sit in peace for 2 to 3 minutes. When you are ready to end your session, bring your hands together in front of your heart, open your eyes, and send gratitude out to the world.

These beginner poses can pack a good punch. They may seem simple, but they are designed to build your mobility, core strength, and balance.

Remember to work at your own rate. This doesn't mean just going through the motions, just to get it finished as quickly as possible!

Listen to your body, and when you feel ready to push on and increase the difficulty level, even if it's just for one set, then do it. If you feel you need to pull back and make it a little easier or take a slightly longer rest between sets, then that's fine as well. Gradual progress is the key to success in any exercise program.

As you practice, keep in mind why you started your chair yoga program and what you want to achieve over the next 21 days. Well done for your hard work.

When you feel ready, move on to the next chapter, where we will work on your intermediate chair yoga routine.

FREE BONUS
DAY 1 – 7 CHAIR YOGA PROGRAM TRACKER

When you begin any exercise program, it's important to keep track of exactly what program you are following and exactly which days you completed it. To help you with this, I have put together your day 1-7 beginner program chart including the images, and a daily tracker to help you to keep on top of it. I have also included a video guide to the whole program as well as the audiobook to make it easier for you to follow.

Go to bit.ly/chair-yoga-free in your internet browser, and I'll forward you the links you need.

You can also scan the QR Code below with your cell phone camera and tap the pop-up link if you find that easier.

I hope that this helps you to get the most out of your chair yoga plan over the next 7 days.

7

INTERMEDIATE CHAIR YOGA PROGRAM DAY 8 - 14

"If it doesn't challenge you, it doesn't change you."

- FRED DEVITO

Once you have progressed through the day 1 to 7 beginner chair yoga program and you feel ready, it is time to move on and start to push your strength, flexibility, and balance to the next level.

As always, take your time to get each pose right, aiming for good form, but never take your movements to the point that it feels painful. You will improve as time goes on. Let's get started with your intermediate chair yoga program.

Days 8 to 14

Prepare Your Body

As you did in your beginner program, run through your dynamic stretches to warm up your muscles and prepare your joints for the exercise. Now sit on your chair in mountain pose and connect with your breath to prepare your mind for the program ahead.

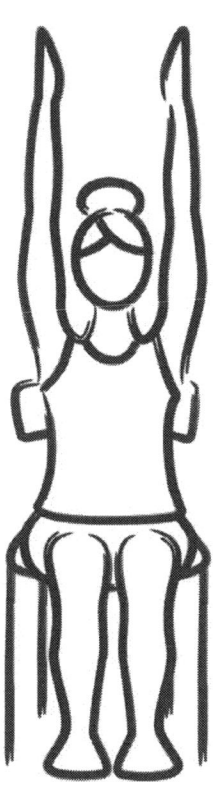

Front Arm Lift

- First, sit upright on your chair and engage your core muscles. Extend both arms in front, with your palms facing each other.
- Inhale and lift both arms overhead, extending your spine and stretching upward. Hold this stretch for 3 to 5 breaths.
- Exhale as you lower both arms back out in front of you.

- Complete 15 to 20 repetitions.
- Rest for 20 to 30 seconds before repeating for 2 more sets.

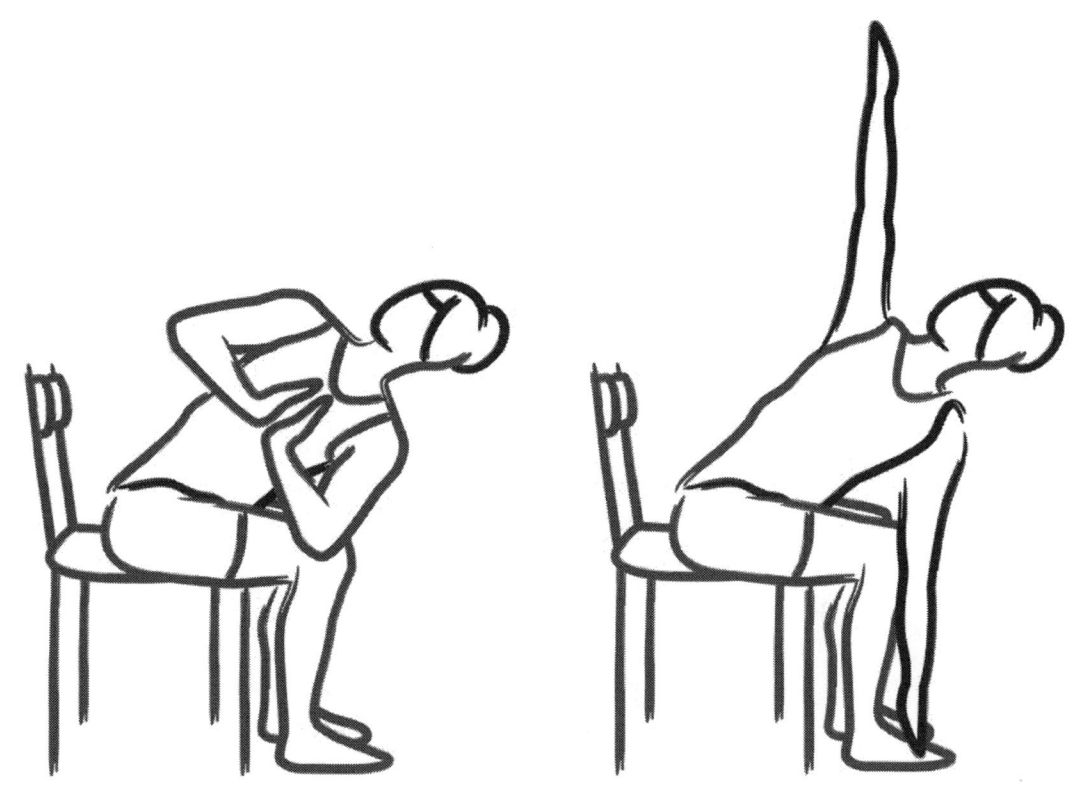

Seated Twist

The seated twist builds both flexion and rotational range in your spine while simultaneously engaging your core muscles, giving focus to your internal and external obliques (they are your side abs). Building and protecting the range in your back helps to reduce or completely release back and neck pain.

To get into a seated twist:

- Start in mountain pose. Keep both feet together, ideally with your big toes touching.

- Inhale and raise the arms above your head like you did in your front arm lift.
- As you exhale, hinge your hips, tipping your body at the waist and reaching the chest towards your thighs. As you move, lower your arms, placing them in a chest-height prayer position. Take a deep breath in.
- Exhaling, twist the torso to the right. Ideally, it should be until your left elbow sits just outside of your right thigh or until you feel a strong but controlled stretch.
- Press the upper left arm against your thigh and draw the right shoulder blade into the back as you turn to the right to increase the stretch if you can. If you can, turn your head towards the ceiling to reach full range. Hold for 5 breaths.
- From this point, you can either recenter your body and repeat on the opposite side, or you can advance to the straight arm version.
- If you are ready to advance to the straight-arm version of the seated twist, extend your left arm, aiming to touch your fingertips on the floor.
- Now, extend your right arm, reaching your fingertips toward the ceiling.
- Hold for another 3 to 5 breaths before returning your arms to a prayer position.
- Now, return to your start position before repeating on the opposite side.
- Complete 3 to 5 repetitions on each side.

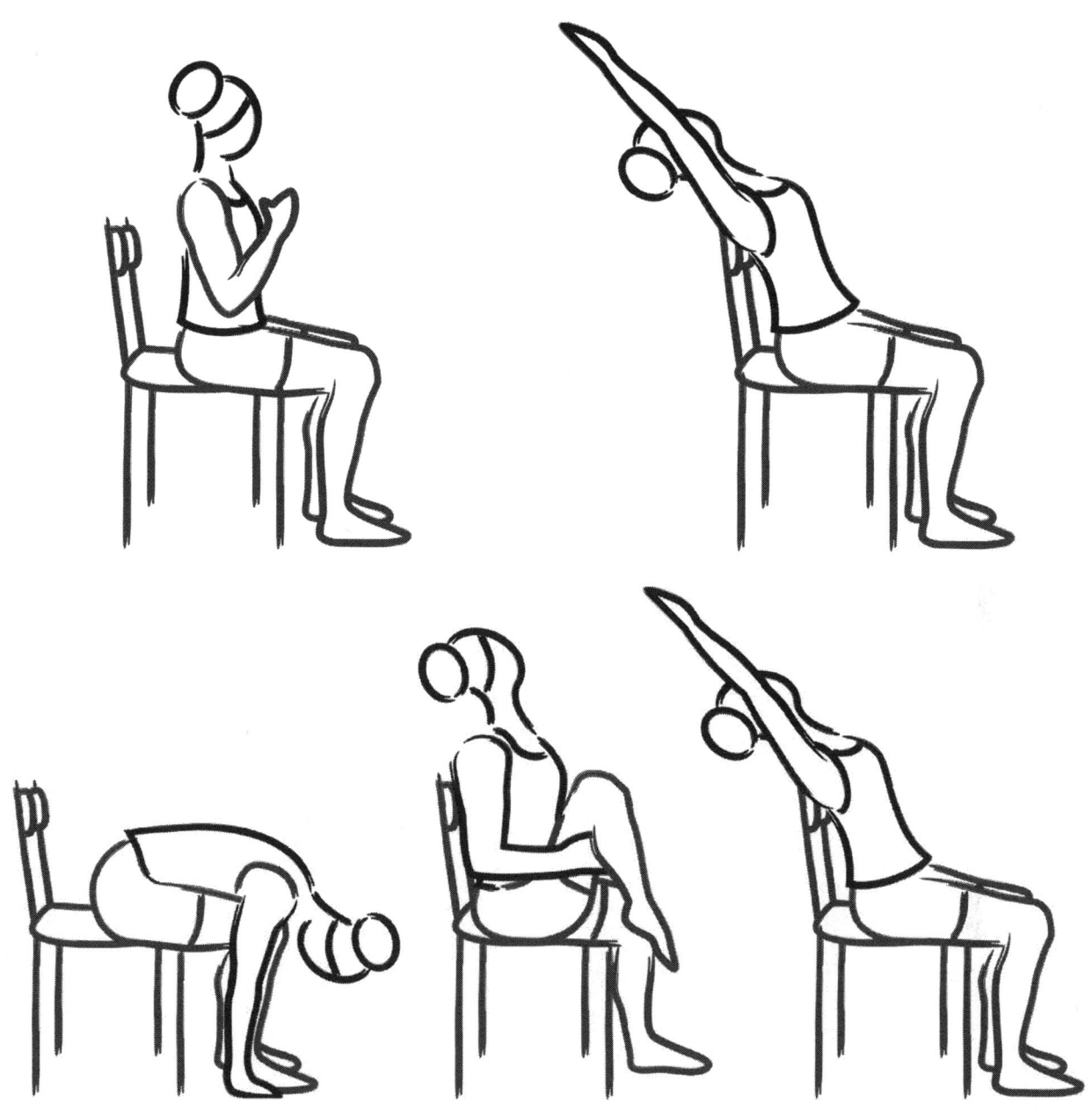

Adapted Sun Salutation

The adapted sun salutation looks almost like a full chair yoga routine in itself. It combines several movements that we have already practiced together, which I will give you refresher teaching points for, with a high knee raise to further improve your hip range and stability.

As you practice the adapted sun salutation, I want you to focus on synching your breath with your movements, breathing in as you release and out as you exert. Concentrate on flowing between movements as smoothly as possible to further build your mind/muscle connection and your overall control.

Let's begin:

- Start in mountain pose, keeping both feet planted on the floor, ideally hip distance apart. Now inhale.
- Exhale and bring the palms together to the front of your chest in a prayer position. Hold for 3 breaths, finishing on an inhale.
- Exhale and raise your arms overhead, leaning against the chair's backrest, and extend your spine. Once at range, gently look your head upward toward the ceiling. Hold position for 3 breaths, finishing on an inhale.
- Exhale and release the stretch. Lower your arms until your hands are on your thighs. Hinge at the hips and fold your body into a full-range forward fold, working to keep the spine and neck long. Slide your hands down your legs and feet, relaxing your neck the entire time until your hands touch the floor. Hold the position for 3 breaths.
- Inhale and rise up, returning to mountain pose. Tuck both hands under your right thigh (just above the knee).
- Exhale and, using your arms, draw your right knee toward your chest. Once you reach your current full range of movement, draw your shoulder blades back and down to expand your chest. Hold the position for 3 breaths.

- Gently lower your leg until your foot is back on the floor. Now inhale.
- Exhale while you reach your arms overhead and extend your spine while leaning against the chair's backrest. Once at range, look upward towards the ceiling. Hold for 3 breaths.
- Exhale and return to mountain pose with your hands in front of your chest in a prayer position. Hold for 3 breaths.
- Repeat a full cycle of the adapted sun salutation, but this time draw your left leg toward your chest.
- Once you have completed a full cycle for both legs, repeat 3 to 5 more times on each side.

There's quite a lot to the adapted sun salutation. The good news is that you have already practiced many of the movements earlier in the book. Learning methods like this that help your chair yoga poses and movements to flow together helps work on your full body strength, mobility, and stability while in motion and is a fantastic way to teach your body to deal with whatever life may throw at it.

CHAIR YOGA FOR SENIORS OVER 60

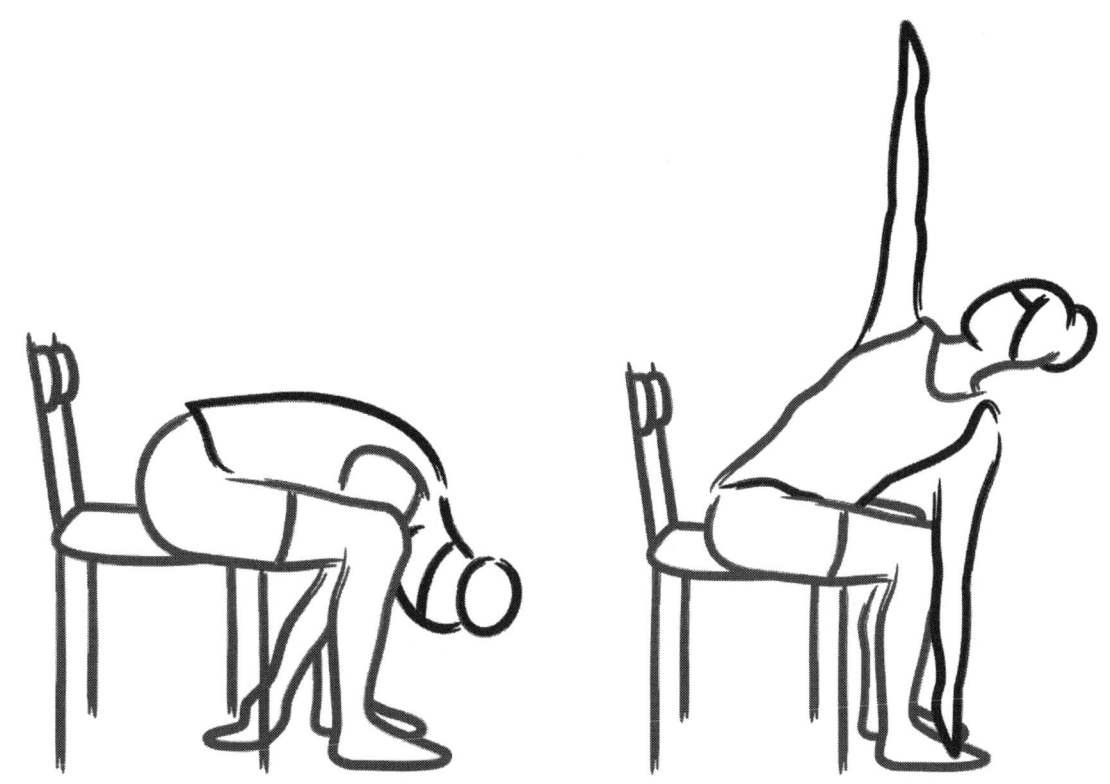

Forward Fold with Twists

This pose combination puts together the full range seated forward fold that we practiced in Chapter 4, with the seated twist that we practiced earlier in this chapter.

Here are the key teaching points to both so you can get right to it:

- Start in mountain pose with your feet at shoulders width apart to begin with. Now breathe in.
- As you exhale, under control, hinge forward at your hips, tipping your body until your chest is either in line with your thighs or as close as comfortably possible.
- Once in position, reach both hands behind you while looking towards your fingertips. Hold for 3 to 5 breaths.

- Return to mountain pose, place your hands in a prayer position in front of your chest, and inhale.
- As you exhale, tip your hips and rotate to your right until you are in a seated twist position. As part of the same movement, slowly extend both arms until your left is touching your right foot and your right is pointed straight overhead. Once in position, turn your head to the right so that you're looking at your right hand. Hold the position for 3 to 5 breaths before returning to a mountain pose.
- Take a moment before repeating the forward fold with twist on the opposite side.
- Repeat 3 to 5 times on each side.

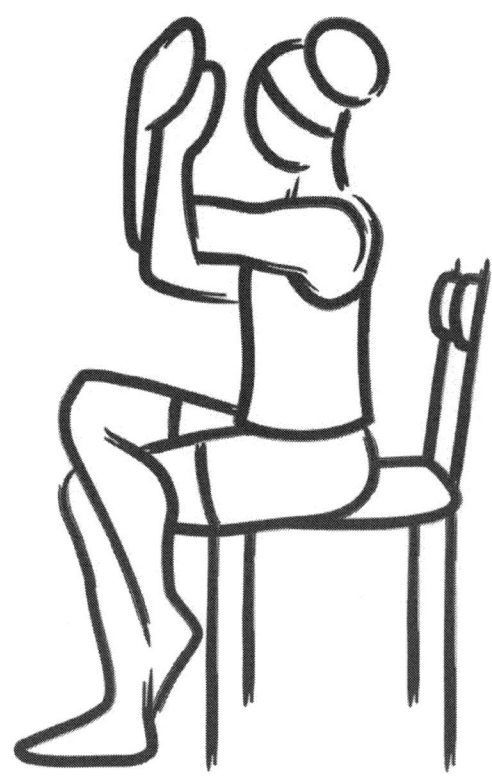

Chair Eagle

Here are the key teaching points for the chair eagle.

- Sit upright in your chair away from its backrest.
- Cross your right thigh over the left, and wind your right foot around the back of your left ankle. If you haven't quite managed to build your range to that point yet, take it to a level that works for you.
- At chest height, cross the left arm over the right. The two arms should meet at the elbow. Bend at the elbows and touch your palms together. If you can't quite make this position, that's not a problem. Push your range as far as you comfortably can. Each time you practice, your range will increase.
- Once in position, hold for 10 breaths before releasing.

- Return to your starting position before repeating on the opposite side.

If you would like a little more detail to refresh your memory, please refer to Chapter 5.

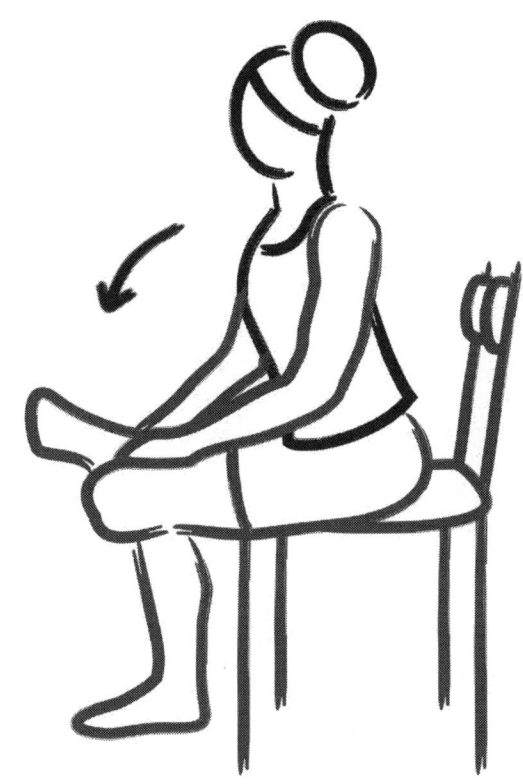

Chair Pigeon

As we've discussed through this book, healthy hip function is absolutely paramount to improving and maintaining an active life. Keeping that in mind, we will focus on further increasing your hip and glute range next with a chair pigeon.

Here are the key teaching points to follow:

- Sit in an upright position, and then cross your left leg over your right, getting into an ankle-to-knee stretch position.
- Once there, gently hinge at your hips to tip your body forward, trying to maintain a strong and straight posture as you do so. This will dramatically increase the stretch in your left glute.
- Once you've found your suitable range, using your left hand on your left knee, gently press down toward the floor. This will help to keep your form strict while further increasing your hip's range. Go easy with this, as it can increase the intensity fast.
- Hold the pain-free stretch position for 10 controlled breaths before releasing and returning to your start position.
- Repeat on the opposite side.

This pose is tough, and you may feel like you're unable to push your range very far to begin with. Don't feel discouraged. Keep in mind that the aim of all these movements and poses is to feel what you're trying to target and to work at your current range with a view to improve a little each time you practice your program. Even if you start off by taking small, consistent steps toward your goal, you are still moving toward it.

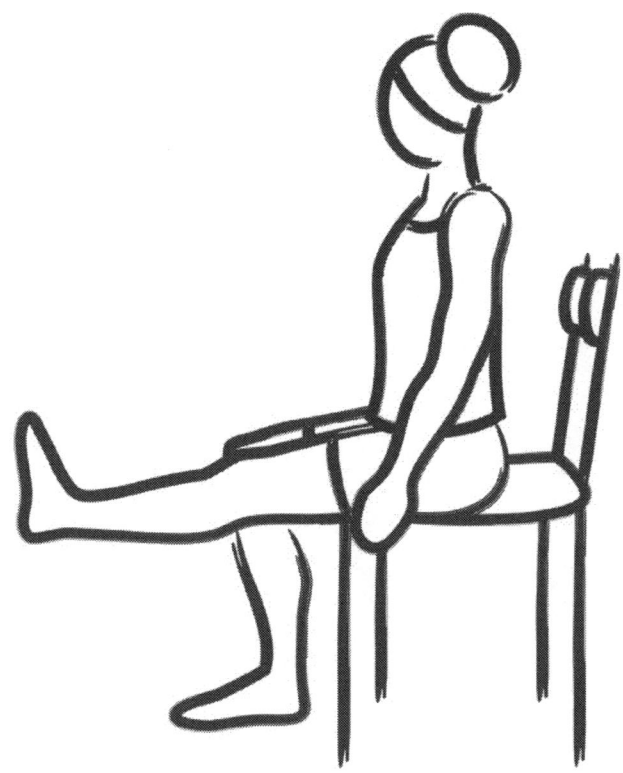

Seated Leg Extension

Next, we are going to focus on building strength in your legs, specifically your quadriceps, and stability in your knees. In the previous chapter, we discussed some of the direct benefits of the seated leg extension. Now that you understand the principles, and hopefully, without sounding too much like a science lesson, I want to touch on something called reciprocal inhibition.

The basics of this are as follows: when you contract (brace or tense) a muscle, your nervous system, which acts as your secondary brain, tells your opposing muscle to relax (switch off). So, in the case of the seated leg extension, when you lift your leg to squeeze your quadriceps (the front of your thigh), your nervous system cleverly signals your hamstrings (the back of your thigh) to relax and lengthen.

This is often used to help alleviate muscle cramps and also to improve a muscle's state of relaxation before it is stretched. This technique applies to your whole body, not just your legs, and I think that now you are working on an intermediate chair yoga program, it's well worth thinking about as you run through your movements.

Here are the key teaching points for a seated leg extension:

- Sit upright in your chair with your feet hip distance apart.
- Place your hands on either side of the seat to help stabilize your position as you move. You can grip the edges of the seat if that works better for you.
- Extend your left leg, lifting your foot upward in front of you until your leg is straight and at the height of your chair's seat for maximum range.
- Hold for 3 breaths before returning your foot slowly to the floor.
- Complete for 10 to 15 repetitions before repeating on the opposite leg.
- Take a 20 to 30 second rest before repeating for another 2 sets on each leg.

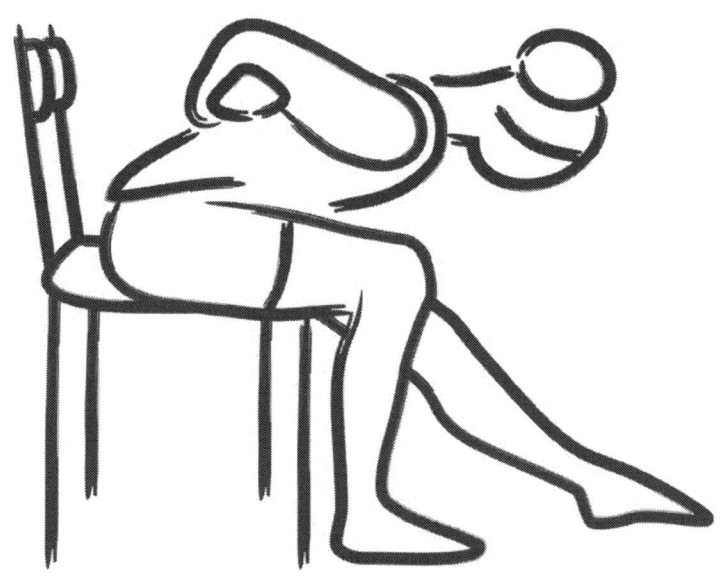

Seated Pyramid

The Seated Pyramid pose combines a forward fold, a leg extension, and a shoulder stretch and is considered high skill. I'm confident that by this stage in your chair yoga journey, you will have the core strength and flexibility to tackle it, so let's get straight to it.

Here are the key teaching points for the seated pyramid pose:

- Sit in an upright position away from your chair's backrest with your feet hip distance apart.
- While keeping your left foot flat on the ground, extend your left leg out in front of you as far as you can while maintaining a good, seated posture.
- Keep your right knee folded at 90 degrees with your right foot flat on the ground.

- Clasp your hands together behind your back and gently push them out behind you until you can feel your shoulders stretching.
- Hinge forward through your hips, drawing your shoulder blades back and down, expanding your chest.
- Once in position, press both feet downwards into the floor to brace your body fully.
- Hold for 5 to 10 breaths before returning to your start position.
- Repeat with your right leg extended.

When you feel ready, here are two simple ways to increase the intensity of this pose.

- With your left leg extended, rather than having your right leg folded to 90 degrees, tuck your right foot under your chair while keeping both feet flat on the floor. This increases the range in your knee and ankle.
- Rather than clasping your hands behind your back, cross your arms behind your back so that you hold your opposite elbow in each hand. This increases the intensity of the pose on your upper body.

These progressions are optional but worth trying once you have practiced the pose and are confident.

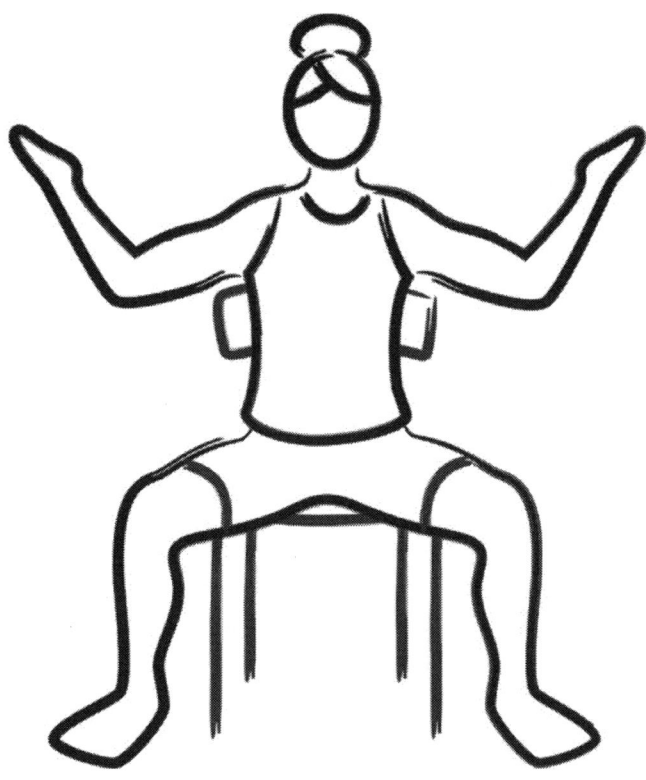

The Goddess

The Goddess is almost the exact opposite of the eagle pose. Its focus is on opening the chest and shoulders while also opening the hip's range by lengthening the adductors (the inner part of your thigh). This pose is both grounding and empowering, especially after all the hard work that you've already put into this program.

Follow the teaching points to get the most out of the Goddess pose:

- Start in mountain pose. Open your hips as wide as you can while splaying your feet.
- Ensure that your knees are directly over your feet for proper alignment. If you have reached your maximum hip range and your knees are falling inward, slightly narrow your stance to correct.

- Once you are in position, lift brace your legs outward until you can feel a strong but controlled stretch.
- Now that your legs are in position, raise both arms laterally (out to your sides) until they are just below shoulder height, with your palms facing up.
- Fold both your arms upward at the elbows until they are at 90 degrees or less.
- Now your arms are in position draw your shoulder blades back and downward while lifting your chest and elongating your neck. Once in the position, you will feel your chest opening outward and your spine extend.
- Now you are in a full Goddess pose, draw your abs inward to fully engage your core muscles.
- Shut your eyes and breathe normally for 15 to 20 breaths before releasing.

While you run through your chair yoga programs, remember to take your time when you transition from one movement to the next. Always focus on smooth control and good form while running through your program at a rate that works for you.

Now that we have completed your intermediate chair yoga program, I recommend that you take a couple of minutes to cool down before continuing with your day.

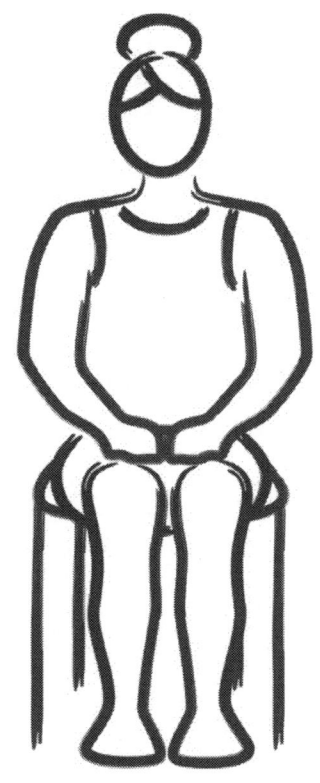

Seated Savasana

Now that you have completed your intermediate chair yoga program, I recommend that you take one or two minutes before continuing with your day. We practiced the seated Savasana at the end of your evening chair yoga program and discussed a visualization method to help you enter a meditative state. In this chapter, I would like to discuss the "why" for this pose, if you need to refresh your memory of the "how," please refer to Chapter 5.

Practicing a seated Savasana for two to three minutes offers many awesome benefits, especially after exercise of any kind. I have listed the key benefits so you can see how something so simple can have such an amazing impact on your body.

5 of the main benefits include:

- Brings calmness and balance to the nervous system, resulting in a positive effect on both the immune system and your digestion.
- It helps to control and, in many cases, can help to reduce blood pressure.
- Helps relax some of the body's trigger points to reduce tension headaches, stress, and fatigue.
- Quiets the mind to help relieve anxiety.
- Promotes clarity of thinking, mindfulness, and awareness of your energy flow.

Every time you run through this program, whatever level you start at, you will further edge your progress forward, and the good news is that it will feel a little easier time.

Stay focused on what you're working to achieve and push yourself enough each day so that you keep improving at a rate that suits your current level.

Some days, it will feel easy, and some days, it will feel tough. An important question to ask yourself on days that you don't feel motivated is, "What kind of life do I want to live?" Your answer should always be "A fully active and independent life."

Well done for making it through the intermediate program. When you're ready to level up again, progress on to the final chapter.

FREE BONUS
DAY 8 – 14 CHAIR YOGA PROGRAM TRACKER

Well done for making it to week 2 of your 21-day chair yoga program. As I mentioned before, it's important to keep track of exactly what program you are following and exactly which days you managed to complete it. To help you stay on target, I have put together a video guide and a full color chart for this stage covering each pose from this program, along with a daily tracker.

Go to bit.ly/chair-yoga-free in your internet browser, and I'll forward you what you need to make it easier to keep on top of the program.

You can also scan the QR Code below with your cell phone camera and tap on the link that pops up if you find that easier.

I hope that this helps you get the most out of your next 7-day program.

8

ADVANCED CHAIR YOGA PROGRAM DAY 15 - 21

"Patience, persistence, and perspiration make an unbeatable combination for success."

- NAPOLEON HILL

Welcome to your advanced chair yoga program! You've already worked hard, making it through your beginner and intermediate programs, which is an incredible achievement. Now it's time to step it up once more and tackle the top-tier program from this book.

So, without further ado, let's get started!

Warm Up

As with your beginner and intermediate programs, please run through your dynamic stretches before you begin your advanced chair yoga program to ensure that your body and mind are properly prepared.

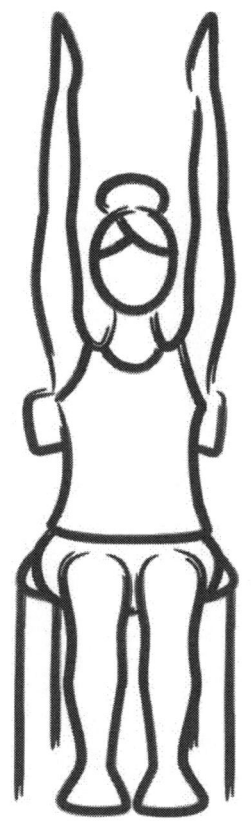

Front Arm Lift

- Sit upright with your feet planted hip width or narrower, slightly forward from your chair's backrest.
- Lengthen your spine and lengthen your neck.
- Draw your shoulders back and down.
- Raise your arms forward and then overhead with your palms facing each other, keeping them shoulder width apart.
- Once your arms are both overhead, look your head upward through the center of your hands while maintaining a strong posture.
- Hold this position for 5 to 10 breaths before lowering your arms.

- Complete 5 repetitions, remembering to synch your breath with your movements.

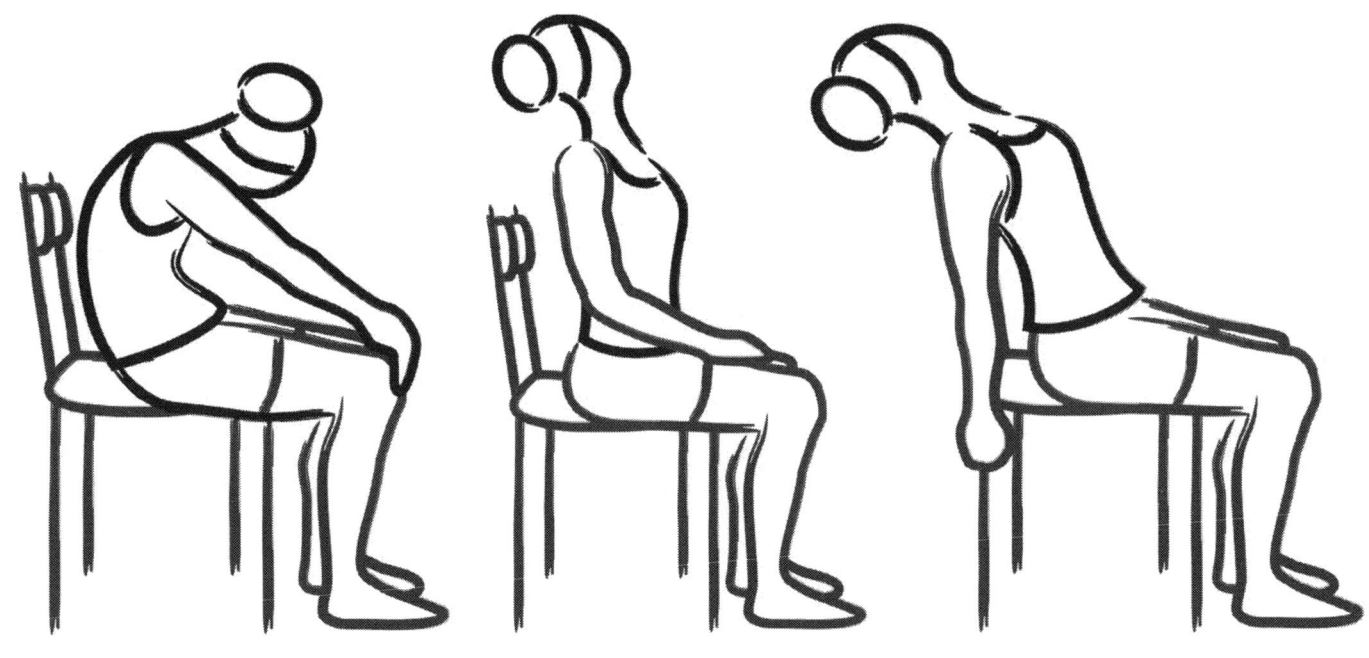

Cat-Cow-Camel

This combination of movements is the same as the seated cat-cow stretch that you practiced in Chapter 2, except this time, it includes an unsupported spine extension in between.

Please follow these key teaching points:

- Sit upright on your chair with your feet hip-width apart (we will refer to this as your neutral position), away from the chair's backrest. Rest your hands on your knees and breathe in.
- As you exhale, grip the front of your knees and round your spine toward the chair's backrest. Drop your chin to your chest and draw in your abs as you do.

- Hold for 3 to 5 breaths before returning to your neutral position.
- From your neutral position, place your hands on your lap and breathe in.
- As you breathe out, draw your shoulders back and downward while lifting your chest toward the ceiling, feeling your spine lengthen. Once at range, lift your chin slightly to extend your neck.
- Hold for 3 to 5 breaths.
- Move your arms to your sides, grip the back of your chair's seat for support and breathe in.
- As you breathe out, fully extend your spine to its end of range. Lift your chin further if possible.
- Focus on keeping your shoulder blades drawn back and down and hold for 3 to 5 breaths. If you need some extra support, allow your upper back to lean against your chair's backrest.
- Exhale and return to your neutral position.
- Repeat for 8 to 10 repetitions.

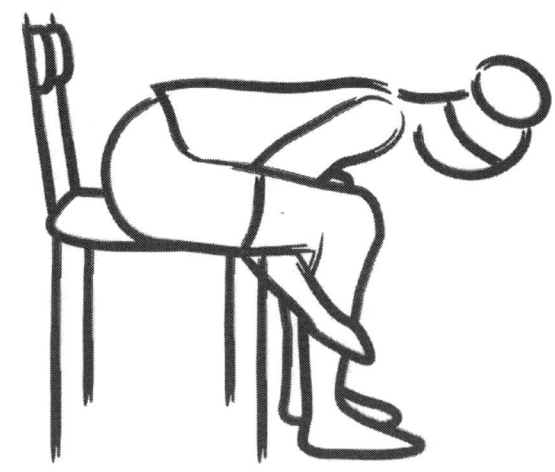

Happy Baby (In a Chair)

Now that you have mobilized your spine, it's time to turn your attention to your hips. Your focus in this pose should be on maintaining posture in your back while increasing the range of movement in your hips.

Here's how:

- Sit in an upright position in your chair, with your feet shoulder width apart, slightly forward from your chair's backrest. Now, breathe in.
- As you breathe out, hinge forward from your hips, tipping your body until you are parallel with the ground.
- Inhale and reach your arms between your legs, winding them outward and around the backs of your calves or ankles.
- Gently pull your torso downward while continuing to maintain a good posture.

- Remember to always work pain-free. That may mean that you must reduce your range to maintain form.
- Hold for 8 to 12 breaths before releasing the stretch and returning to an upright seated position.

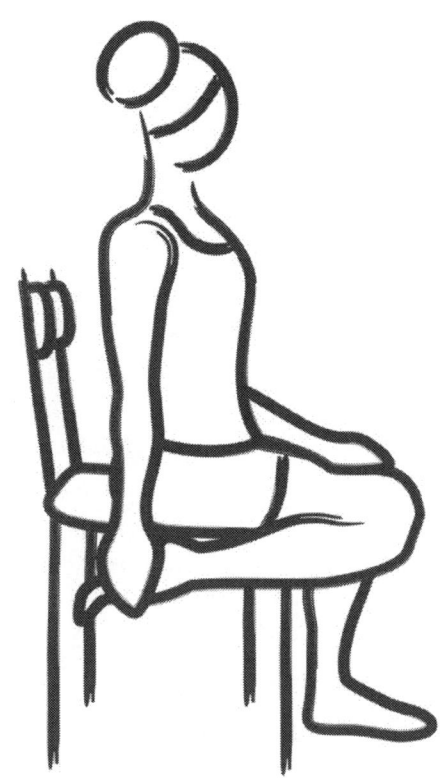

King Arthur's Pose

King Arthur's pose focuses on proprioception (this means your body's ability to correct itself without conscious thought), core stability, as well as knee and ankle range of movement. A big part of living an independent life comes down to how quickly you can correct your footing if something goes wrong.

Note:

Core stability and proprioception go hand in hand. Training your proprioception teaches your nervous system to make quick corrections before you even realize there's a problem.

The ultimate demonstration of this is a tightrope walker on a high wire. They are constantly correcting their balance faster than they can think to stop them from falling. Now, I'm not suggesting that you set up a tightrope in your living room, but I think it illustrates proprioception well.

To practice the King Arthur's pose, follow these teaching points:

- Sit upright on the right side of your chair, slightly away from the back rest, with your feet hip distance apart.
- Brace your body, focusing on keeping your hips level and your left foot planted on the ground.
- Bend your right knee until your foot has lifted off the floor. Reach down with your right arm and gently pull your foot towards your hips while pointing your toes.
- When you are in position, I want you to focus your attention on your left knee. Make sure that it is not falling inward. If it has, gently push it outward until it's in line with your left foot.
- Once you are in alignment, lift your chest and draw your shoulder blades back and down to complete the pose. You will notice that, as well as a stretch through your right thigh, this position is incredibly unstable, making it a challenge to hold. This is where your proprioceptive muscles and core stability come into action. Breathe normally, draw in your abs, and hold form for up to 30 seconds or as long as you comfortably can.

- If you can't hold for the full 30 seconds. I would like you to break the set down into smaller chunks of time that add up to around the full 30. Just place your foot down to balance when you take a rest.
- Once you have completed your set, relax the position, take 20 seconds rest, and then practice the pose on your opposite side.

If you found this pose to be particularly tough on your balance, that's a sure sign that you need it! The good news is that proprioception improves fast. Just like how your muscle tone develops, all the improvements happen after the set is complete, and your body takes a moment to understand and learn from the overload that has been placed upon it.

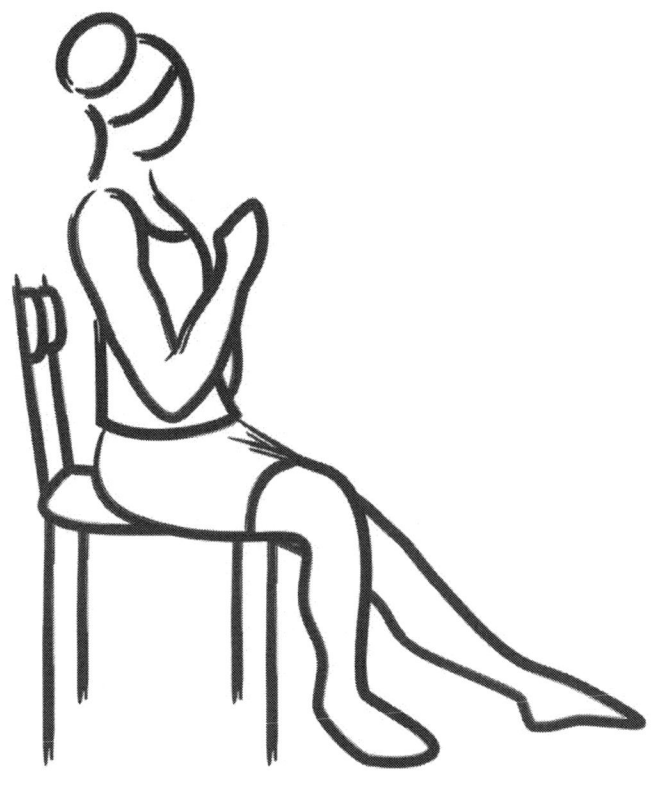

The Tree Pose

The tree pose is especially good for helping strengthen and build range in your knees and ankles. It works well with the previous pose, and once you are confident with both, you can flow between them or use them as stand-alone.

The teaching points for the tree pose are as follows:

- Sit upright, slightly forward on your chair, with your feet hip distance apart and your hands in a prayer position in front of your chest.
- Inhale deeply, lift your chest and then exhale as you draw your shoulder blades down and back. Look straight ahead.

- Extend your left leg straight out in front of you, pointing your toes forward with your foot flat on the floor.
- While keeping your right knee at 90 degrees, allow it to hang outward while keeping your foot flat on the floor. Now inhale.
- As you exhale, stretch your arms overhead into a front arm lift position and hold for 3 to 5 deep breaths.
- When ready, exhale and bring your arms back to a prayer position in front of your chest.
- Switch your leg position and practice the pose on the opposite side.
- Repeat for 5 repetitions on each side.

Take a rest between repetitions if needed.

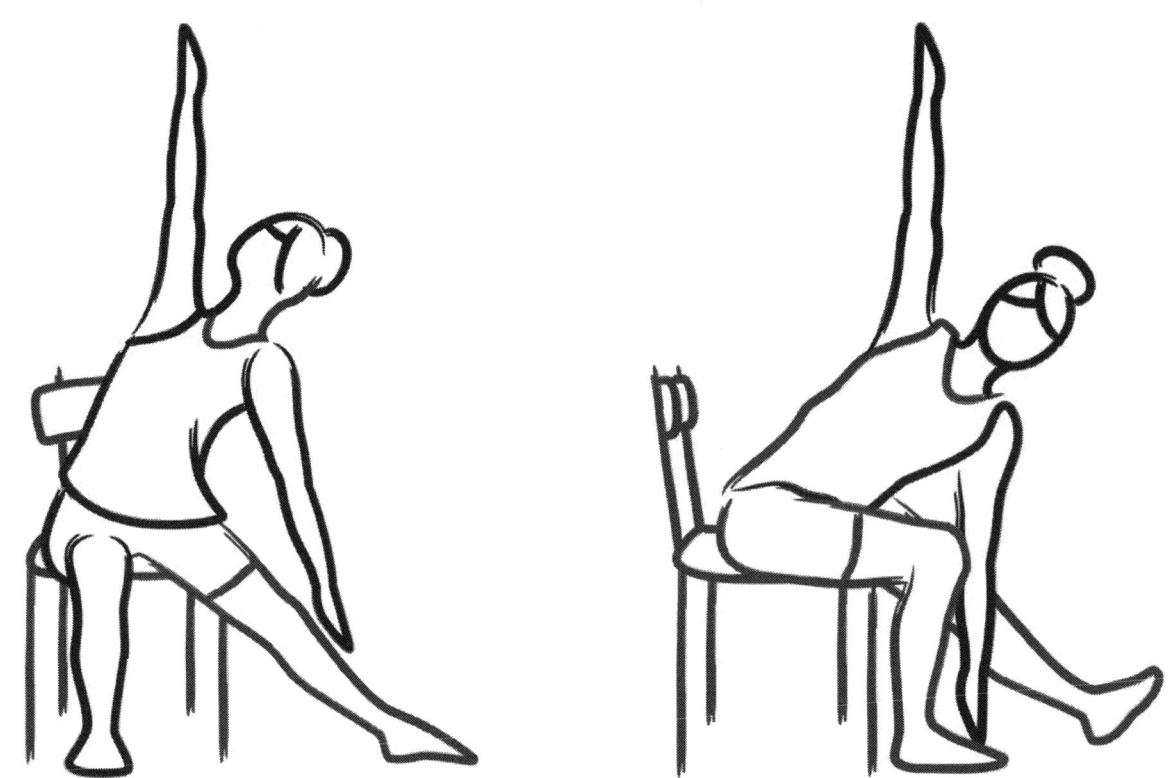

Extended Triangle Pose

The extended triangle pose combines several of the other movements that we have already practiced together. Take your time and follow the teaching points to get the most out of it.

- Sit upright to the left side of the chair, ideally with your left thigh slightly off the chair's seat.
- Keeping your right leg routed to the floor, extend your left leg out straight at the knee and out at a left angle at the hip. Once you are in position, brace your thigh.
- Inhale and raise both arms to shoulder height laterally (to the sides) with your chest open, holding them parallel to the floor. Keep your shoulder blades drawn back, and your palms face down.

ADVANCED CHAIR YOGA PROGRAM: DAY 8 - 14

- Exhale and lean your torso to the left, aiming your left hand toward your outstretched left leg's knee or shin. As you reach downward with your left arm, reach upward with your right, rotating your right palm up and aiming toward the ceiling. Once in position, turn your head until you can see your right fingertips.
- Hold this position for 8 to 10 breaths.

From this point, if you feel this is as far as you can take this position today, return to your starting position before practicing it on the opposite side.

If you feel ready to advance further, please continue on the same side with the following teaching points.

- Breathe in.
- As you breathe out, keep your right arm reaching upward and your left arm straight, rotate your torso to the right, aiming to touch your right foot with your left hand.
- Turn your head from looking upward to looking straight.
- Hold the position for 8 to 10 breaths before returning to your start position and repeating both extended triangle pose positions on the opposite side.
- Take 20 to 30 seconds rest before repeating for 2 to 4 more sets on each side.

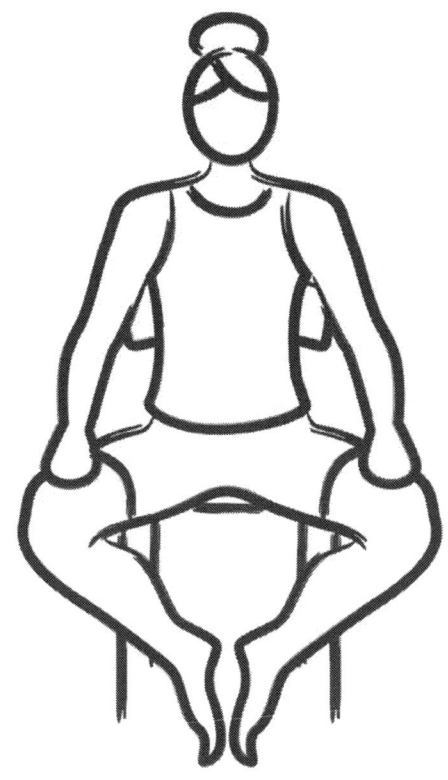

Bound Angle Pose

Similar to the Garland pose we practiced in Chapter 3, the bound angle pose opens your hips range, lengthening your adductors (inner thighs) and groin in the process. Improving and maintaining a good range of rotational movement in the hips helps to protect both your knees and your lower back. Some of the other benefits the bound angle pose offers include stimulating your abdominal organs and improving your circulation.

- Sit upright to the front of your chair with your feet narrow. This gives your legs space to move while seated.
- Come up onto the balls of your feet, and then move your knees apart as far as your current range will allow.

- Place your hands on your knees and breathe in.
- As you breathe out, gently increase the stretch by pushing your knees outward with your hands. As you do this, draw your shoulder blades back and down, lengthening your spine and neck.
- Hold for 8 to 10 breaths before releasing the stretch and returning to your start position.
- Repeat for 2 to 4 more sets.

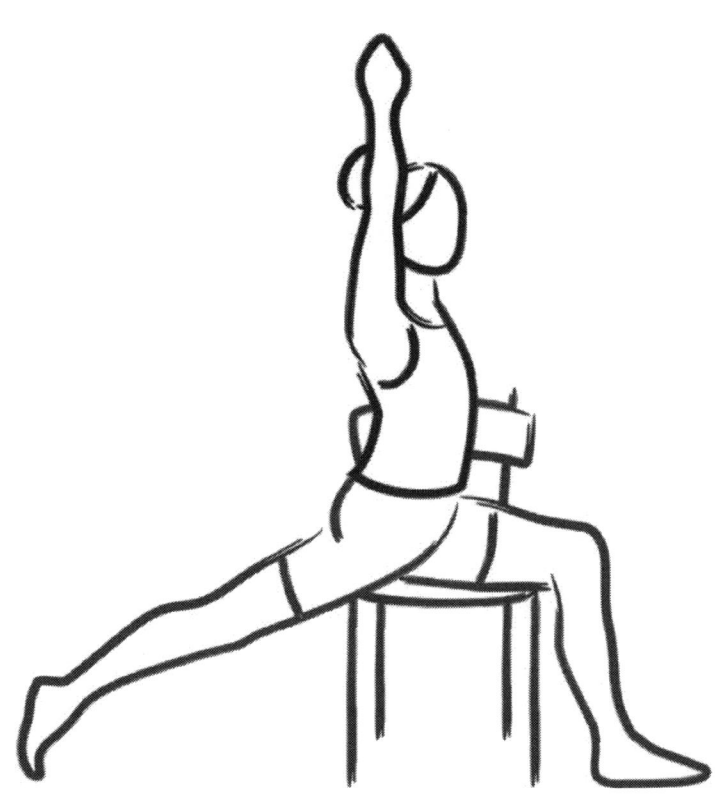

Seated High Lunge

Similar to the various chair warrior poses that we practiced earlier in this book, the seated high lunge will challenge your flexibility, strength, and balance all at once. One of the main focuses of this pose is the position of your hips. The key to getting the most benefits from this pose is to keep your hips facing forward to properly load and lengthen your hip flexors. I will run you through the teaching points in a moment, but before I do, I wanted to highlight this. Its other benefits include toning and strengthening your thighs, knees, ankles, and core.

- Sit sideways on your chair so that its backrest is next to your left arm. Sit toward the edge of the chair so that your left thigh is supported and your right has space to move.
- Hold onto the top of the chair's backrest with your left hand to help support you through the position.
- Keeping your left foot planted on the floor in front of you with its knee at 90 degrees, lengthen your right leg out behind you, perching on the ball of your right foot. You are now in a basic high lunge position.

If this is as far as you can take it today. Hold for 5 to 10 breaths before repeating on the other side.

If you would like to advance the position, please continue.

- From this position, bring attention to your hips. As I mentioned earlier, the key to this pose is to ensure that your hips are square to the way that you're facing, so gently adjust until you feel a strong but pain-free stretch in the front of your right hip.
- Once your hips are in position, I want you to turn your attention to your right foot. Sometimes, the heel will fall in toward your center line. If possible, push your heel outward until your foot is exactly upright and facing forward. Now, take a breath in.

- As you breathe out, reach your right arm upward, toward the ceiling with your palm facing in, and lengthen your spine.
- Hold for 5 to 10 breaths before releasing the stretch and switching to the opposite side.
- Repeat 2 to 3 more times on each side, taking a 30-second rest between sets.

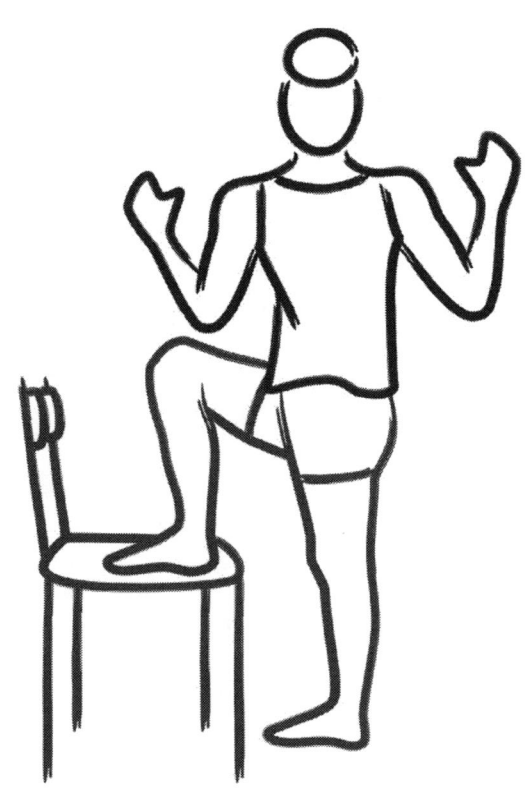

Marichyasana 3

As well as improving your hip function, your spine's rotation, and your ability to use your glutes to balance, the marichyasana 3 pose is considered to detoxify the body by gently massaging both your kidneys and liver. Like with any twisting movement, take your time to build your range and balance. I recommend that you start off with your chair next to a wall so you have something to brace against while you practice.

The following teaching points will walk you through it:

- Place your chair next to a wall and stand facing it, with your right shoulder next to the wall.
- Keeping your left foot on the floor and facing forward, place your right foot onto the chair's seat. Keep your right hand on the wall for balance. Take a breath in.
- As you breathe out, rotate to your right, towards the wall, placing both hands on the wall wider than shoulder distance apart and at chin height.
- Turn your head to the right until you are at your maximum range, and draw your shoulder blades back and down.
- If you would like to increase your range, use your arms to gently pull you further around to the right, remembering not to force it.
- Focus on your left leg and the support it's giving you, while drawing your abs in to activate your core muscles.
- Now, bring your focus to your left glute, bracing it as you hold to reinforce your mind/muscle connection. This will help to teach your glutes to strengthen your balance when on one leg.
- Hold the position for 10 breaths before returning to your start position, and repeating on the opposite side.
- Once you have completed a set on both sides, take a 20 to 30 seconds rest and repeat for 2 to 3 more sets on each side.

ADVANCED CHAIR YOGA PROGRAM: DAY 8 - 14

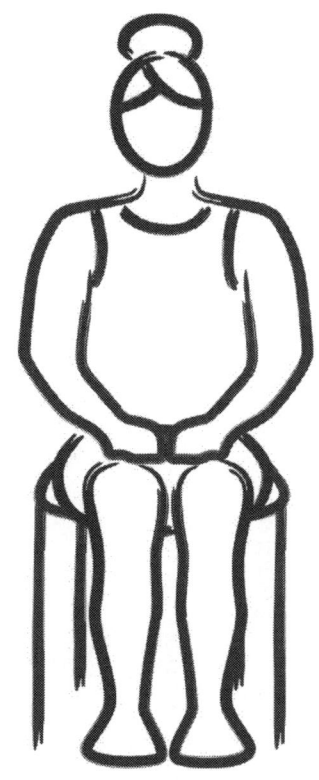

Seated Savasana

In this program, you have pushed yourself hard through some tough chair yoga movements and poses. I recommend finishing your session today with 2 to 3 minutes of seated savasana to allow your mind and body to recover before you continue with your day.

FREE BONUS
DAY 15 – 21 CHAIR YOGA PROGRAM TRACKER

You've made it through to the 3rd week of your 21-day chair yoga program. Amazing work! You should be starting to notice an improvement in your flexibility, your stability, and your overall chair yoga skill level as you run through each of the poses.

To help you stay motivated and on track, I have put together a full video guide along with a useful chair yoga pose chart, and a daily tracker to help you complete your day 15-21 advanced chair yoga program.

To access this free download, type bit.ly/chair-yoga-free into your internet browser, and I'll send you what you need.

You can also scan the QR Code below with your cell phone camera and tap on the pop-up link if you find that easier.

I hope that this helps keep you motivated and on target over the last 7 days of your 21-day program, and a big well done to you for staying the course!

Before We Conclude Our Journey Together

I have a question to ask you: Would you be willing to help me if all it cost you was less than 60 seconds of your time?

If you would, that's fantastic news! All you have to do is leave an honest review for this book on Amazon.

Even though the simple act of leaving a review will take you less than 60 seconds, it will give a huge amount of support.

It may help one more senior citizen to live the life of independence that they want. Perhaps it will help one more person reduce their daily pain. It may help to improve one more over 60's life for the better.

To make that happen and to keep it quick and simple, scan the QR code below that corresponds to you with your cell phone camera, and press the link that pops up to go directly to your Amazon review page:

Review Amazon US

Review Amazon UK

Review Amazon CA	Review Amazon Worldwide

If you don't want to click on a link, you can head to your Amazon orders page, locate this book, scroll down just below where the reviews are listed, and click the 'Write a review' option.

Thank you from the bottom of my heart for your time. You have just made my day.

Anyway, on with the show.

- Your coach, Arthur

CONCLUSION

In this guide, my goal has been to teach you more than just a handful of chair yoga poses. I wanted to teach you their purpose too. What you should be feeling when you practice. What some of the technical mumbo-jumbo actually means and how to apply it correctly. How to adapt each movement to suit you, and how these movements and poses can greatly reduce pain and discomfort, improve your mobility, balance, and strength, and help you keep living an active life.

You have also learned how to activate your core muscles and the importance of keeping them strong and stable, how to drive your body's movements correctly and under total control to dynamically build your range of motion, and how and why to train your proprioception to ensure that you are always stable on your feet.

To finish our chair yoga journey together, we went through a progressive 21-day program covering three skill levels, progressing from beginner, to intermediate, to advanced, giving you the option to repeat the programs that work best for your current level for 21 days or follow each for 7 days before progressing to the next.

All the poses and programs we have worked on together have been specially designed to improve your overall strength and stamina, your balance and stability, your flexibility and controlled range of movement, and ultimately, your ability to live a pain-free, strong, and independent life. It's crazy to think that such wonderful goals can be achieved simply by exercising while seated in a chair and without the need for a gym or any special equipment.

I'm extremely proud of you for making it through the book, and I'm even prouder that you chose me to be your coach. If you'd like to get in touch to tell me about your chair yoga success, I'd love to hear all about it. You can reach me at arthur@expertchairyoga.com.

Stay focused, practice consistently, and believe that you can achieve your goals. You now have all the tools you need to improve your balance, strength, and mobility in just 21 days.

Healthy regards,

Arthur

References

10 Yoga Poses You Can Do in a Chair. (n.d.). Verywell Fit. https://www.verywellfit.com/chair-yoga-poses-3567189

30 Minute Chair Yoga Sequence. (2019, September 10). Purple Lotus Yoga. https://www.purplelotusyoga.com/30-minute-chair-yoga-sequence/

ademarsh. (2019, December 29). *Accessible Yoga: Chair Sun Salutation.* Yoga Journal. https://www.yogajournal.com/practice/chair-sun-salutation/

admin. (2022, March 31). *Guide to the Perfect Yoga Warm Up Routine.* Yoga for Beginners | Beginners Yoga | Yoga School in India. https://yogaforbeginners.yoga/guide-to-the-perfect-yoga-warm-up-routine/#:~:text=The%20Benefits%20of%20Yoga%20Warm%20Up%201%201.

REFERENCES

Ashish. (2022, May 18). *The Way of Yogic Breathing: How to Breathe Correctly During Yoga.* Fitsri. https://www.fitsri.com/articles/yogic-breathing-how-to-breathe-during-yoga

Bedosky, L. (2022, May 17). *The 10 Best Chair Exercises For Seniors.* Get Healthy U | Chris Freytag. https://gethealthyu.com/best-seated-exercises-for-seniors/#:~:text=How%20to%20perform%20a%20seated%20side%20bend%3A%201

Bedtime Yoga: Benefits and Poses to Try. (2020, June 17). Healthline. https://www.healthline.com/health/healthy-sleep/bedtime-yoga

Cleveland Clinic. (2020, May 29). *Understanding the Difference Between Dynamic and Static Stretching.* Health Essentials from Cleveland Clinic. https://health.clevelandclinic.org/understanding-the-difference-between-dynamic-and-static-stretching/

Francis. (2023, May 16). *The Benefits of Doing Yoga in the Morning - Healing Picks.* https://healingpicks.com/the-benefits-of-doing-yoga-in-the-morning/

How to Do a Leg Extension: Techniques, Benefits, Variations. (n.d.). Verywell Fit. Retrieved October 19, 2023, from https://www.verywellfit.com/leg-extensions-benefit-or-risk-3498573#:~:text=For%20a%20seated%20leg%20extension%20with%20ankle%20weights%2C

How to perform the Hip Circles - Physitrack. (n.d.). Www.physitrack.com. Retrieved October 19, 2023, from https://www.physitrack.com/exercise-library/how-to-perform-the-hip-circles-exercise#how-to-perform

McGonigle, A. (2022, August 22). *5 Ways to Practice Pyramid Pose.* Yoga Journal. https://www.yogajournal.com/practice/5-ways-to-practice-pyramid-pose/#Pyramid%20Pose%20in%20A%20Chair

Mellardo, A. (2023, September 11). *5 Easy Chair Yoga Exercises for Beginners.* Eat This Not That. https://www.eatthis.com/chair-yoga-

REFERENCES

exercises-for-beginners/#:~:text=5%20Easy%20Chair%20Yoga%20Exercises%20for%20Beginners%201

Rony. (2018, July 9). *My 8 tips to progress in yoga.* Speaky Magazine. https://www.speakymagazine.com/my-8-tips-to-progress-in-yoga/

Use This Gentle Chair Yoga for Seniors Routine to Reduce Pain & Anxiety. (n.d.). Dr. Axe. Retrieved October 19, 2023, from https://draxe.com/fitness/chair-yoga-for-seniors/#Best_Gentle_Chair_Yoga_for_Seniors_Routine_12_Minutes

Washington, A. (2013, October 7). *The Importance Of Focus in Yoga (And Life).* DoYou. https://www.doyou.com/the-importance-of-focus-in-yoga-and-life/

Why are hip exercises so important? (n.d.). Bare Biology. https://www.barebiology.com/blogs/news/why-are-hip-exercises-so-important

Why Is Breath So Important in Yoga? (2013, December 30). DoYou. https://www.doyou.com/why-is-breath-so-important-in-yoga/

Made in the USA
Columbia, SC
16 March 2024

33155304R00119